Men's Health Unlocked:

A Guide to Living Well

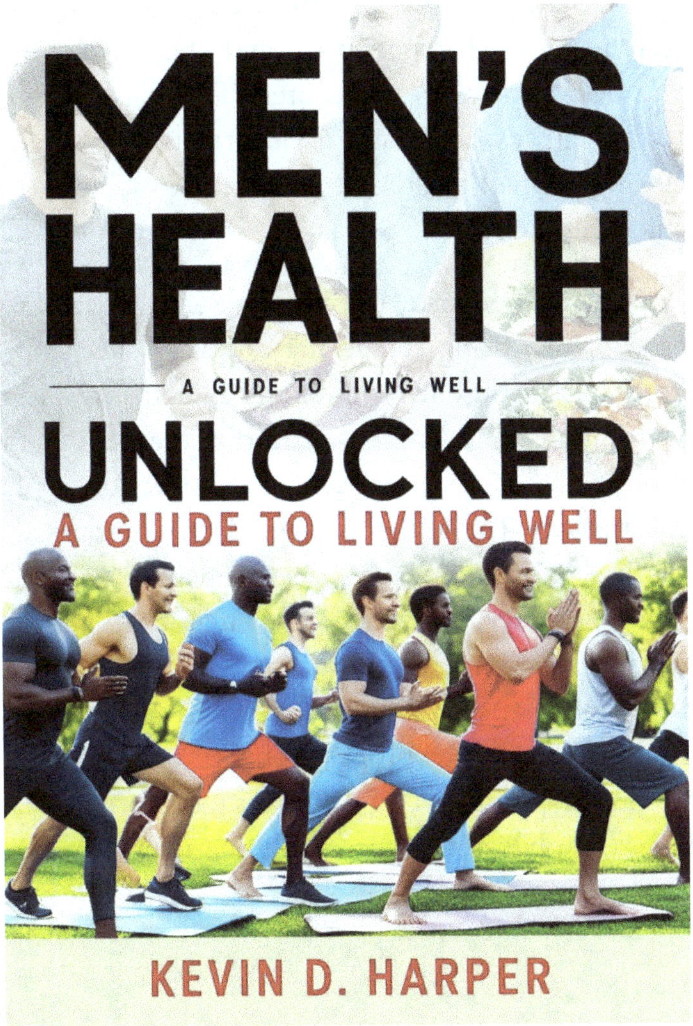

Copyright © by Kevin D. Harper

No part of this book may be reproduced, stored in a retrieval system, or transmitted in any form or by any means, electronic, mechanical, photocopying, recording, or otherwise, without the prior written permission of the author, except for brief quotations used in critical reviews or scholarly works. This book is a work of nonfiction intended to provide general information and guidance on health, fitness, and wellness for men. The advice and strategies presented in this book are based on the author's research, personal experiences, and the collective insights of experts in the field. However, the content is not intended to replace professional medical advice, diagnosis, or treatment. Readers should always consult a qualified healthcare provider for advice regarding any health or medical condition.

While every effort has been made to ensure the accuracy and reliability of the information in this book, the author and publisher cannot be held responsible for any errors or omissions or any outcomes resulting from the use of this information. The content reflects the author's opinions and experiences as of the publication date and may not apply to every individual or situation. The author and publisher encourage readers to approach health and wellness with a personalized, holistic mindset, considering diet, exercise, mental well-being, and lifestyle choices. Tailoring health strategies to one's own unique needs and circumstances is essential. All trademarks, registered trademarks, and product names mentioned in this book are the property of their respective owners. Any references to specific products or brands are for informational purposes only and do not imply endorsement or affiliation with the author or publisher.

Introduction

Welcome to Men's Health Unlocked: A Guide to Living Well, your essential roadmap to achieving optimal health, well-being, and longevity. Whether you're looking to improve your fitness, sharpen your mind, or build lasting habits, this book will guide you every step of the way. Inside, you'll discover proven strategies and practical insights explicitly designed for men to live healthily.

Why This Book Matters

In today's fast-paced world, men often put their health on the back burner. Work, family, and social obligations can easily overshadow the need for proper self-care. However, making time for your health is one of the most important investments. Men's Health Unlocked offers a fresh, no-nonsense approach to health and wellness tailored to men's unique needs.

What You Will Learn

In this book, we will cover the following key areas to help you transform your health and live well:

- **Building a Balanced Routine:** Simple, actionable strategies to improve your fitness and nutrition without feeling overwhelmed.
- **Mental and Emotional Well-being:** Techniques for reducing stress, improving mental clarity, and achieving emotional balance.
- **Lifestyle Habits for Longevity:** Insights into how everyday habits, from sleep to social connections, impact your long-term health.
- **Overcoming Common Health Barriers:** Solutions to common challenges men face, including weight management, heart health, and muscle building.

What Makes This Book Different

Unlike generic health advice, Men's Health Unlocked is designed with your unique goals. Whether you're just starting your journey or looking to refine your current routine, this guide provides:

- **Real-life strategies** based on the latest research.
- **Personal stories** and examples from men who have successfully transformed their health.
- **Practical tips** you can easily integrate into your busy life.

Now is the time to unlock your best health.

By taking the first step today, you'll be on the path to a stronger, more energetic, and balanced version of yourself. It's time to prioritize health because you deserve to live well.

Table of Contents

Chapter 1: Understanding Men's Health

1.1 Overview of Men's Health Statistics and Common Issues

Men's health has been a topic of growing concern in the past few decades, with particular attention being drawn to disparities in health outcomes between men and women. Globally, men have a shorter life expectancy than women, and they tend to suffer from a range of health problems at higher rates. This chapter provides a comprehensive look at the health challenges faced by men, supported by relevant statistics and an understanding of the most common issues impacting their well-being.

1.1.1 Life Expectancy and Mortality Rates

On average, men have a shorter life expectancy compared to women. According to the World Health Organization (WHO), men's average life expectancy is around 70 years, while women typically live around 76 years. This difference is partly due to biological factors such as hormones, but lifestyle choices, risk factors, and healthcare access also influence it.

The disparity is even more pronounced in many countries, particularly in low and middle-income regions. Men are also more likely to die prematurely from preventable causes such as accidents, violence, and lifestyle-related diseases.

1.1.2 Leading Causes of Death Among Men

The leading causes of death among men vary based on region, age, and socioeconomic factors. However, some of the most prevalent causes of mortality worldwide include:

- **Cardiovascular Diseases**: Heart disease is the leading cause of death among men globally. Men are more likely to develop heart disease at an earlier age compared to women, and lifestyle factors like high-fat diets, sedentary behavior, smoking, and alcohol consumption contribute significantly to this trend.
- **Cancer**: Various forms of cancer, including prostate, lung, and colorectal cancer, are among the most common causes of death for men. Prostate cancer, in particular, is the second most common cancer worldwide and significantly affects older men.
- **Diabetes**: Type 2 diabetes is another growing concern among men. It is primarily influenced by obesity, poor diet, and lack of physical activity, leading to complications such as heart disease, kidney failure, and amputations.
- **Respiratory Diseases**: Chronic obstructive pulmonary disease (COPD) and other respiratory diseases are more common in men, particularly among smokers. These conditions contribute significantly to premature death.
- **Accidents and Injuries**: Men are more likely to be involved in fatal accidents and injuries, whether due to risky behaviors like driving under the influence, workplace accidents, or physical confrontations.

1.1.3 Mental Health and Suicide Rates

Mental health is critical to overall health, yet it is often overlooked in men's health discussions. Men are less likely to seek help for mental health issues and more likely to engage in harmful coping behaviors such as substance abuse or aggression. Depression, anxiety, and stress are prevalent, but they are often underreported, and many men may not receive the necessary support due to societal stigma.

Suicide rates are significantly higher in men, particularly in middle-aged and older men. Men are three times more likely than women to die by suicide. The pressures of financial responsibility, work-related stress, and relationship difficulties are contributing factors.

1.1.4 Reproductive and Sexual Health

Men's reproductive health is another area of concern. Issues such as erectile dysfunction (ED), low testosterone, and infertility are often left untreated due to embarrassment or lack of awareness. The stigma surrounding these issues prevents many men from seeking medical advice or treatment, leading to adverse effects on their quality of life and relationships.

Sexual health disorders, including sexually transmitted infections (STIs), are also significant health concerns for men. Safe sexual practices are essential for preventing the spread of diseases, but many men fail to use protection, particularly in high-risk populations.

1.2 Importance of Addressing Men's Health Specifically

While many health issues affect both men and women, addressing their health precisely due to their unique challenges is essential. Ignoring these differences can result in missed opportunities to improve overall health outcomes for men, reduce healthcare disparities, and promote better quality of life. Addressing men's health can be broken down into several key reasons.

1.2.1 Tailored Prevention and Treatment Strategies

Men's health requires specific, tailored prevention and treatment strategies considering their biological, psychological, and social needs. For instance, men are more likely to engage in risky behaviors such as smoking, excessive drinking, and physical inactivity. Public health initiatives focused on reducing these behaviors and encouraging healthier lifestyles can profoundly impact reducing preventable health conditions among men.

Moreover, the healthcare system often fails to consider men's unique medical needs. For example, prostate cancer screening is crucial for men over 50, but it is frequently underutilized due to a lack of awareness or reluctance to undergo testing. Tailored education campaigns and targeted healthcare services are vital for addressing these concerns effectively.

1.2.2 Socioeconomic and Cultural Factors

Socioeconomic and cultural factors also play a significant role in men's health. In many cultures, there is a prevailing notion that men should be stoic and resilient, often resulting in the suppression of emotional and physical needs. Men are usually less likely to seek medical attention due to fear of appearing weak or vulnerable. These cultural norms prevent men from accessing the care they need and contribute to the worsening of chronic conditions.

Additionally, men in lower socioeconomic brackets may experience higher rates of preventable diseases, partly due to reduced access to healthcare services, unhealthy living conditions, and financial instability. Focusing on addressing these inequalities is crucial in improving men's health outcomes.

1.2.3 Early Detection and Health Screening

Early detection is key to successfully treating many health conditions, and men are less likely to undergo regular screenings and check-ups than women. For example, routine screening for colorectal cancer, prostate cancer, and cardiovascular conditions is often underutilized by men. Raising awareness about the importance of early detection and making screenings more accessible can significantly reduce the disease burden in men.

1.2.4 Gender-Specific Mental Health Needs

Men have specific mental health needs that often go unaddressed. Traditional masculinity norms may discourage men from expressing vulnerability, making it harder for them to reach out for support when facing mental health challenges. Providing mental health services and outreach programs tailored to men can help reduce stigma and improve the overall well-being of male populations.

1.3 The Impact of Societal Norms on Men's Health Behaviors

Societal norms play a crucial role in shaping health behaviors, and for men, these norms often have a negative impact on their health outcomes. The expectations placed on men to be strong, self-reliant, and emotionally stoic can deter them from seeking medical help, engaging in preventive care, or addressing emotional distress.

1.3.1 The Culture of Masculinity

The culture of masculinity, which values traits such as toughness, independence, and emotional restraint, has a profound effect on how men perceive their health. Many men are socialized to believe that seeking help for physical or mental health problems is a sign of weakness. This cultural attitude has significant consequences, particularly in the context of mental health, where men are more likely to deny symptoms of depression or anxiety and avoid seeking help.

Furthermore, the pressure to conform to masculine ideals can lead to risky behaviors. For example, many men may feel compelled to engage in dangerous activities such as excessive drinking or risky driving to demonstrate their toughness or resilience. These behaviors not only pose significant health risks but can also lead to long-term physical and psychological harm.

1.3.2 The Role of Media and Advertising

Media and advertising contribute to reinforcing harmful masculine stereotypes. Advertisements often portray men as being invulnerable, self-sufficient, and aggressive, which further perpetuates the stigma surrounding vulnerability and health issues. For instance, the portrayal of idealized male bodies in the media can lead to unrealistic expectations and body image issues, especially in younger men. This can contribute to unhealthy behaviors such as excessive dieting, steroid use, or extreme physical training to achieve an idealized body.

1.3.3 The Impact on Health-Seeking Behavior

The societal pressure for men to be "tough" can prevent them from seeking medical care when needed. Men are less likely to visit doctors for preventive care, and when they seek help, it is often when a condition has already progressed to a more severe stage. As a result, diseases like cancer, heart disease, and diabetes are usually diagnosed at later stages, reducing the likelihood of successful treatment.

Moreover, men are more likely to use alcohol, tobacco, and other substances as coping mechanisms to deal with stress, which can have detrimental effects on both mental and physical health.

1.3.4 Mental Health Stigma

Mental health issues, especially those involving depression, anxiety, or emotional distress, are often considered taboo in many societies. Men who experience mental health struggles are less likely to reach out for help, fearing judgment or rejection. This stigma prevents open discussions about mental health and creates a barrier to treatment. Encouraging a shift in how mental health is perceived within the context of masculinity is essential for improving the mental well-being of men.

Conclusion

Understanding men's health is crucial to addressing the health disparities between men and women. Men face unique challenges in their health that are often exacerbated by societal norms, which discourage them from seeking help or discussing their health openly. By recognizing the importance of men's health and addressing the specific factors that influence their health behaviors, it is possible to improve the health outcomes for men and promote a more equitable approach to healthcare. Through education, targeted interventions, and a shift in cultural norms, society can better support men in leading healthier lives.

Chapter 2: The Foundation of Physical Fitness

1. **Benefits of Regular Exercise for Men**

Physical fitness is crucial for overall health and well-being. When done consistently, exercise offers a wide range of benefits, especially for men. These advantages span from improved mental health to reduced risk of chronic diseases and enhanced physical performance. Below are some of the primary benefits of regular exercise for men.

1. **Improved Cardiovascular Health**

Regular exercise helps strengthen the heart muscle, improve circulation, and lower blood pressure. It is particularly important for men at higher risk for heart disease. Cardiovascular exercises such as running, cycling, and swimming help reduce cholesterol levels, improve blood vessel function, and promote better heart health overall. Studies have shown that men who engage in consistent physical activity have a significantly reduced risk of heart disease and stroke.

1. **Weight Management**

Exercise plays a central role in weight management. By increasing caloric expenditure through physical activity, men can maintain a healthy body weight or reduce excess fat. Strength training, in particular, helps increase lean muscle mass, which boosts the metabolic rate, making it easier to maintain a healthy weight. Regular exercise promotes weight loss, especially with a balanced diet.

1. **Enhanced Muscular Strength and Endurance**

Strength training is one of the most beneficial types of exercise for men, mainly because it builds muscle mass, increases strength, and enhances overall endurance. As men age, they naturally experience a decline in muscle mass, but regular resistance training can counteract this. Improved muscular strength makes day-to-day activities easier and improves posture, flexibility, and overall physical performance.

1. **Mental Health Benefits**

Exercise has profound effects on mental health, reducing symptoms of anxiety, depression, and stress. Regular physical activity releases endorphins, which are natural mood lifters. For men, maintaining mental well-being is just as important as physical health, and exercise is one of the most effective ways to manage mental health issues. Additionally, engaging in group fitness classes or team sports can foster social connections and support networks, which are crucial for emotional health.

1. **Increased Energy Levels**

One of the most immediate benefits of regular exercise is boosting energy levels. Contrary to the belief that exercise makes you tired, physical activity increases the body's energy production systems, helping men feel more energized throughout the day. This is especially important for busy men who juggle work, family, and social commitments.

1. **Reduced Risk of Chronic Diseases**

Regular exercise lowers the risk of chronic diseases such as type 2 diabetes, high blood pressure, and certain cancers. For example, men who engage in physical activity regularly have a much lower risk of developing type 2 diabetes because exercise improves insulin sensitivity. Additionally, men who exercise frequently show a decreased risk of prostate and colorectal cancers.

1. **Improved Longevity and Quality of Life**

Exercising regularly helps to promote a longer, healthier life. Men who live an active lifestyle tend to have a better overall quality of life and are less likely to experience chronic pain, disability, and age-related decline. Furthermore, regular physical activity contributes to maintaining cognitive health, improving memory, and reducing the risk of dementia.

1. **Types of Exercises: Strength Training, Cardio, Flexibility**

Exercise can be broadly categorized into three main types: strength training, cardiovascular (cardio) exercises, and flexibility training. Each type uniquely enhances physical fitness and should be incorporated into a balanced fitness routine. Below is an in-depth exploration of each exercise type.

1. **Strength Training (Resistance Training)**

Strength training, also known as resistance training, involves exercises that target specific muscles using resistance, either through weights, machines, or body weight. The primary goal of strength training is to build muscle, increase bone density, and improve joint function.

- **Benefits**: Strength training helps men increase muscle mass and strength. It also promotes fat loss, as muscle burns more calories at rest than fat. Moreover, strength training effectively improves bone density, which can help prevent osteoporosis later in life. It can be performed using free weights (dumbbells, barbells), machines, or bodyweight exercises (push-ups, squats).
- **Common Exercises**: Squats, deadlifts, bench presses, bicep curls, lunges, and rows are some of the most common strength exercises. Compound movements (exercises that target multiple muscle groups at once), like squats and deadlifts, are particularly effective for building muscle and strength.
- **Frequency**: Strength training should be done 2-4 times per week, with at least one rest day between workouts to allow the muscles to recover and grow.

1. **Cardio (Aerobic Exercise)**

Cardiovascular or aerobic exercise is any form of exercise that increases the heart rate and improves the efficiency of the heart and lungs. Cardio exercises are essential for overall heart health and fat burning.

- **Benefits**: Cardiovascular exercise improves endurance, helps burn calories, and improves heart health. It is also effective for managing weight, reducing the risk of chronic diseases like heart disease, and promoting healthy blood circulation. Cardio exercises enhance the body's ability to use oxygen efficiently and boost overall stamina.
- **Common Exercises**: Running, cycling, swimming, rowing, and hiking are common forms of cardio. High-intensity interval Training (HIIT) is another popular form of cardio that alternates between short bursts of intense activity and recovery periods.
- **Frequency**: Ideally, men should aim for at least 150 minutes of moderate-intensity aerobic activity (like brisk walking or swimming) or 75 minutes of vigorous-intensity activity (like running or cycling) per week.

1. **Flexibility Training (Stretching and Mobility)**

Flexibility training involves exercises that improve the range of motion of muscles and joints, reduce muscle stiffness, and prevent injuries.

- **Benefits**: Stretching increases flexibility, reduces the risk of muscle strains and injuries, and promotes better posture. It also helps in relieving tension and stress. Flexibility training can improve athletic performance by allowing muscles to move freely and efficiently.
- **Common Exercises**: Two common forms of stretching are static stretching (holding a stretch for 20-30 seconds) and dynamic stretching (moving the muscles through a full range of motion, such as leg swings). Yoga and Pilates are also excellent for improving flexibility and mobility.
- **Frequency**: Flexibility exercises should be done daily, particularly after strength or cardio workouts, to help muscles recover and maintain flexibility.

1. **Creating a Balanced Workout Routine**

A well-rounded workout routine incorporates strength training, cardio, and flexibility exercises to address all aspects of physical fitness. A balanced routine can help prevent overtraining in one area while promoting overall health. Here are some steps to creating an effective, balanced workout routine.

1. **Set Clear Goals**

Before starting any workout program, it is essential to define personal fitness goals. These could relate to weight loss, strength gain, muscle toning, endurance, or improving flexibility. Setting clear and measurable goals helps guide the structure of the workout routine and keeps motivation high.

1. **Plan Your Week**

A balanced workout routine should include a combination of strength training, cardio, and flexibility exercises spread throughout the week. For example:

- **Strength Training**: Aim for at least 2-4 sessions per week, focusing on different muscle groups each day. A split workout (e.g., upper body on Monday, lower body on Wednesday) can ensure each muscle group gets the attention it needs.
- **Cardio**: Aim for at least 3-5 weekly cardio sessions, varying the intensity and type to keep things interesting. For instance, you could run or cycle on one day and swim or take a HIIT class on another day.
- **Flexibility**: Incorporate flexibility exercises 5-7 days a week, after workouts or as a separate session. Yoga or Pilates classes can be excellent ways to improve flexibility and build core strength.

1. **Rest and Recovery**

Rest is an essential component of any fitness routine. Overtraining can lead to injury and burnout. Schedule at least 1-2 days of rest or active recovery (light walking, stretching, or yoga) to allow your body to recover and rebuild.

1. **Nutrition and Hydration**

Nutrition plays a vital role in supporting a balanced workout routine. Ensure you're consuming enough protein for muscle repair, carbohydrates for energy, and healthy fats for joint and brain health. Staying hydrated is also critical, especially when engaging in intense physical activity.

1. **Consistency and Progression**

Finally, consistency is key to seeing long-term results. Stick to your routine, progressively challenge yourself (by increasing weights, reps, or cardio intensity), and adjust based on how your body responds.

Conclusion

The foundation of physical fitness is built on a combination of exercise types, each offering unique benefits. Regular exercise, whether strength training, cardio, or flexibility, is crucial for maintaining optimal health, improving physical performance, and enhancing quality of life. A balanced workout routine that includes all these elements is essential for achieving overall fitness and ensuring long-term well-being.

Chapter 3: Nutrition Essentials for Men

Nutrition is essential to overall health and well-being, especially for men, who have unique nutritional needs influenced by factors such as age, physical activity levels, metabolism, and health status. Proper nutrition is not just about eating; it's about fueling the body with the correct nutrients to enhance physical performance, improve mental health, prevent chronic diseases, and maintain optimal body composition. This chapter will explore key nutrients and their roles in men's health, the distinction between macronutrients and micronutrients, and practical meal-planning strategies that promote healthy eating habits.

Key Nutrients and Their Roles in Men's Health

Men's nutritional needs are shaped by several factors, including their larger muscle mass, typically higher calorie needs, and increased metabolism compared to women. Specific nutrients are pivotal in maintaining these physical features and supporting overall health. Below are the key nutrients men need to prioritize:

1. **Protein**

Protein is vital for muscle repair, growth, and maintenance. It is essential for men, as they generally have more muscle mass than women, which requires more protein to support recovery from physical activities. Additionally, protein plays a role in hormone production (including testosterone), immune function, and enzyme production.

- **Sources:** Lean meats, poultry, fish, eggs, dairy, legumes, and plant-based protein sources like tofu, tempeh, quinoa, and lentils.

1. **Carbohydrates**

Carbohydrates are the body's primary source of energy. For men, carbohydrates fuel high-intensity physical activities and are essential for maintaining mental clarity and overall energy levels. They are broken down into glucose, which is then utilized by the muscles and brain.

- **Sources:** Whole grains (brown rice, quinoa, oats), starchy vegetables (sweet potatoes, squash), fruits, and legumes.

1. **Fats**

Fats are crucial for hormonal balance, particularly for testosterone production, which significantly impacts men's muscle mass, metabolism, and overall health. Healthy fats also contribute to brain function, joint health, and the absorption of fat-soluble vitamins (A, D, E, and K).

- **Sources:** Avocados, olive oil, nuts and seeds, fatty fish (salmon, mackerel, sardines), and flaxseeds.

1. **Vitamins and Minerals**

Vitamins and minerals are essential for various bodily functions, including immune health, bone density, energy production, and antioxidant defense. The following are particularly important for men's health:

- **Vitamin D:** Supports bone health, immune function, and mood regulation. It also plays a role in testosterone levels.
  - **Sources:** Sunlight, fortified foods, fatty fish, egg yolks, and mushrooms.
- **Magnesium:** Important for muscle function, sleep regulation, and heart health. Magnesium also helps maintain a healthy blood pressure.
  - **Sources:** Leafy greens, nuts, seeds, whole grains, and legumes.
- **Zinc is essential** for immune health, wound healing, and healthy testosterone levels.
  - **Sources:** Meat, shellfish, beans, seeds, nuts, and whole grains.
- **B vitamins (e.g., B12, B6, and Folate)** Support energy production, brain function, and red blood cell formation.
  - **Sources:** Meat, poultry, fish, eggs, dairy, and fortified cereals.
- **Calcium:** Vital for bone health, muscle function, and nerve transmission.
  - **Sources:** Dairy products, fortified plant-based milk, leafy greens, tofu, and almonds.

1. **Water**

Water is a vital nutrient, critical for hydration, digestion, nutrient transportation, temperature regulation, and detoxification. Due to their higher muscle mass and larger body size, men generally need more water than women.

- **Sources:** Water, fruits, vegetables, and beverages like herbal teas.

1. **Fiber**

Fiber is essential for digestive health, cardiovascular function, and regulating blood sugar levels. It also provides satiety and helps maintain a healthy weight.

- **Sources:** Whole grains, fruits, vegetables, legumes, and seeds.

Understanding Macronutrients and Micronutrients

To build a solid foundation for good nutrition, it is essential to distinguish between macronutrients and micronutrients. Both are critical to health but serve different functions in the body.

Macronutrients

Macronutrients are nutrients the body requires in large amounts because they provide the energy necessary for daily activities. These include protein, carbohydrates, and fats.

1. **Proteins (4 calories per gram)**
    - **Function:** Proteins comprise amino acids, the building blocks of muscle tissue, enzymes, hormones, and immune system components. They are crucial for repairing and growing body tissues and producing enzymes and hormones.
    - **Recommended Intake for Men:** Generally, men should aim to consume about 0.8-1.0 grams of protein per kilogram of body weight daily. This could increase to around 1.2-2.0 grams per kilogram of body weight for active individuals or those aiming to build muscle mass.

2. **Carbohydrates (4 calories per gram)**
    - **Function:** Carbohydrates are the body's preferred energy source. Once digested, they are broken down into glucose and used for energy. Complex carbohydrates, which are rich in fiber, are digested slowly and provide sustained energy.
    - **Recommended Intake for Men:** Carbohydrates should comprise around 45-65% of total daily calories, focusing on complex carbs such as whole grains, fruits, and vegetables.

3. **Fats (9 calories per gram)**
    - **Function:** Fats are essential for hormone production, brain function, and the absorption of fat-soluble vitamins. Healthy fats support cardiovascular health and are a key energy source during prolonged exercise.
    - **Recommended Intake for Men:** Fats should make up around 20-35% of total daily calories. Healthy fats, such as omega-3 fatty acids, should be prioritized over trans fats and saturated fats.

Micronutrients

Micronutrients are vitamins and minerals needed in smaller amounts but just as essential for overall health. They are involved in numerous bodily functions, including enzyme reactions, immune defense, and tissue repair.

1. **Vitamins**
   - **Fat-Soluble Vitamins (A, D, E, K):** These vitamins are stored in the body's fat tissues and liver. They play roles in vision, bone health, immune function, and skin health.
   - **Water-soluble vitamins (B-vitamins, Vitamin C):** These vitamins are not stored in the body and need to be replenished regularly through food. They are involved in energy production, immune health, and wound healing.
2. **Minerals**
   - **Microminerals (Calcium, Magnesium, Potassium, Sodium):** These minerals are required in more significant amounts and support functions such as bone health, muscle function, and nerve transmission.
   - **Trace Minerals (Zinc, Iron, Copper, Iodine):** These are required in smaller amounts but are equally important in maintaining healthy metabolism, immune function, and antioxidant protection.

Meal Planning and Healthy Eating Habits

Adopting healthy eating habits and learning how to plan meals effectively are essential for maintaining optimal nutrition. A balanced diet enhances physical performance, mental clarity, and long-term health.

1. **Creating Balanced Meals**

Each meal should contain a balance of macronutrients to provide sustained energy and essential micronutrients to support bodily functions.

- **Protein:** Incorporating a protein source in every meal helps repair muscle tissue and keeps you full for longer. Examples include lean meats, fish, tofu, eggs, and beans.
- **Carbohydrates:** Choose complex carbohydrates for lasting energy and fiber. Whole grains, legumes, vegetables, and fruits should be regular components of your diet.
- **Healthy Fats:** Don't avoid fats; opt for monounsaturated and polyunsaturated fats such as avocados, nuts, seeds, and fatty fish.

1. **Portion Control**

Maintaining portion control is key to preventing overeating, especially when it comes to high-calorie foods. Aim to consume appropriate portions that align with your energy needs based on your age, activity level, and health goals.

- **Tip:** Use smaller plates and pay attention to hunger cues rather than eating out of habit or boredom.

1. **Meal Timing**

While the timing of meals is a matter of preference, eating regular meals and snacks can help maintain energy levels throughout the day. Avoid skipping meals to prevent overeating later.

- **Tip:** If you're trying to build muscle or improve athletic performance, consuming protein-rich meals spaced evenly throughout the day can support muscle repair and growth.

1. **Hydration**

Proper hydration is an often-overlooked aspect of nutrition. Men should aim to drink at least 3.7 liters (125 ounces) of fluids daily, though this requirement may increase with physical activity or exposure to hot climates.

- **Tip:** Carry a water bottle throughout the day to remind yourself to stay hydrated.

1. **Mindful Eating**

Mindful eating involves paying attention to your food—how it looks, tastes, and feels. This approach can help you identify hunger cues, prevent overeating, and improve digestion.

Conclusion

Proper nutrition is crucial for maintaining health, improving performance, and preventing disease.

Chapter 4: Managing Stress and Mental Well-Being

Introduction

Mental and physical health are intricately linked, and the well-being of one often influences the other. Over the years, the importance of managing stress has gained increasing attention as the world faces fast-paced living, environmental stressors, and a growing awareness of mental health challenges. This chapter delves into the connection between psychological and physical health, explores various techniques for stress management, and provides guidance on recognizing signs of mental health issues.

1. The Connection Between Mental Health and Physical Health

The relationship between mental and physical health is bidirectional, meaning that mental health can directly affect physical health, and physical health can also influence mental well-being. The human body and mind function as a system where an imbalance in one area can ripple through the other.

1.1. The Impact of Mental Health on Physical Health

Stress, anxiety, depression, and other mental health disorders can lead to various physical health problems, including:

- **Cardiovascular Diseases**: Chronic stress has been shown to increase the risk of heart disease, high blood pressure, and stroke. This is due to releasing stress hormones like cortisol and adrenaline, which can raise blood pressure and heart rate. Over time, this can lead to plaque buildup in arteries and increase the risk of heart attack and stroke.

- **Weakened Immune System**: Chronic stress weakens the immune system by suppressing the activity of immune cells like T-cells, which protect against infection. Stress can increase susceptibility to colds, flu, and other illnesses.

- **Digestive Issues**: Stress has a profound effect on the gastrointestinal system, causing issues like irritable bowel syndrome (IBS), heartburn, indigestion, and bloating. Stress can interfere with the normal functioning of the digestive tract, leading to gastrointestinal discomfort.

- **Muscle Tension and Pain**: Stress can cause muscles to tighten, leading to tension and pain, particularly in the neck, shoulders, and back. Chronic muscle tension can contribute to long-term pain and conditions like tension headaches or migraines.

- **Sleep Disorders**: Mental health conditions like anxiety and depression often interfere with sleep patterns. Poor sleep can negatively affect the body, including a weakened immune system, impaired cognitive function, and an increased risk of chronic illnesses.

1.2. The Impact of Physical Health on Mental Health

Physical health problems, on the other hand, can also negatively affect mental well-being. Chronic physical illnesses such as diabetes, cancer, or chronic pain can lead to feelings of hopelessness, anxiety, and depression.

- **Chronic Illness and Depression**: Long-term illnesses can trigger or exacerbate mental health conditions like depression. The uncertainty of dealing with a chronic disease, along with the physical limitations it brings, can contribute to a sense of loss of control, isolation, and emotional distress.

- **Pain and Mental Health**: Chronic pain, especially conditions like arthritis or back pain, is often associated with mental health issues. People in constant pain may experience heightened levels of stress, frustration, and depression. This can create a cycle where pain leads to poor mental health, which in turn exacerbates the pain.

- **Fatigue and Cognitive Decline**: Chronic physical illness can lead to persistent fatigue, affecting cognitive function, concentration, and memory. This mental fog can make it harder to perform daily activities, leading to frustration and, in some cases, a sense of helplessness or depression.

1.3. The Mind-Body Connection

The mind-body connection is the understanding that the mental state directly impacts physical health. Thoughts and emotions trigger various physiological responses in the body. For instance, stress can activate the autonomic nervous system, releasing stress hormones that affect the heart, lungs, muscles, and digestive system.

Additionally, relaxation techniques such as deep breathing, meditation, and mindfulness can activate the parasympathetic nervous system, counteracting the stress response and promoting physical relaxation. When we focus on improving mental health, we often see significant improvements in physical health.

1. Techniques for Stress Management: Mindfulness, Meditation, and Exercise

Effective stress management is essential to maintaining mental and physical well-being. Several techniques, including mindfulness, meditation, and exercise, can help individuals manage stress. These methods promote relaxation, improve emotional regulation, and improve overall mental well-being.

2.1. Mindfulness

Mindfulness is the practice of focusing on the present moment non-judgmentally. It involves fully knowing what is happening around and within you, including thoughts, feelings, and physical sensations, without reacting or becoming overwhelmed.

- **Benefits of Mindfulness**: Numerous studies have shown that mindfulness can reduce stress, enhance emotional regulation, and improve cognitive function. Mindfulness can help individuals become more aware of their stress triggers, allowing them to respond calmly and composedly rather than reacting impulsively.
- **Mindfulness Techniques**: Mindfulness can be practiced in many forms, such as mindful breathing, mindful eating, or simply being present at the moment during daily activities. For instance, focusing on the sensation of your breath as you inhale and exhale or noticing the textures and flavors of food as you eat can help anchor your mind in the present.
- **Mindfulness-Based Stress Reduction (MBSR)**: MBSR is a structured program that reduces stress and promotes well-being through mindfulness practices. It combines mindfulness meditation, body awareness, and gentle yoga to improve mental and physical health. Research has shown that MBSR can significantly reduce symptoms of anxiety, depression, and chronic pain.

2.2. Meditation

Meditation is a mental exercise that involves focusing the mind and eliminating distractions. It can take many forms, including concentrative meditation, loving-kindness meditation, and guided imagery. Meditation promotes relaxation, reduces stress, and enhances overall mental well-being.

- **Types of Meditation**: There are various forms of meditation, each with its focus and technique:
    - **Focused Attention Meditation** involves concentrating on a single object, sound, or thought to calm the mind. For

example, one might focus on the breath, a mantra, or a candle flame.

- **Loving-kindness meditation** Focuses on developing compassion and love toward oneself and others. This practice can enhance emotional well-being and reduce negative emotions like anger or resentment.
- **Guided Meditation**: Involves listening to a recording or a teacher who guides you through a visualization or relaxation exercise. This is particularly helpful for beginners who may struggle to meditate independently.

- **Benefits of Meditation**: Meditation has been shown to reduce symptoms of anxiety, depression, and insomnia. It helps regulate emotions, improves concentration, and enhances the ability to cope with stressful situations. Regular meditation is also linked to lower blood pressure, reduced inflammation, and a more muscular immune system.

2.3. Exercise

Exercise is one of the most effective and scientifically supported methods for reducing stress and improving mental health. Physical activity stimulates the production of endorphins, which are natural mood elevators that can help reduce feelings of anxiety, depression, and stress.

- **Benefits of Exercise**:
  - **Physical Health Benefits**: Regular physical activity improves cardiovascular health, strengthens the immune system, boosts energy levels, and promotes overall physical well-being.
  - **Mental Health Benefits**: Exercise has been shown to reduce symptoms of depression and anxiety, increase self-esteem, and improve cognitive function. It also helps alleviate stress by promoting relaxation and improving sleep quality.
- **Types of Exercise for Stress Management**:
  - **Aerobic Exercise**: Activities such as walking, jogging, cycling, or swimming that elevate the heart rate are highly effective for reducing stress. Aerobic exercise helps improve mood and reduce anxiety by increasing the release of neurotransmitters like serotonin and dopamine.

- **Strength Training**: Weightlifting and resistance exercises also offer stress-reducing benefits. These exercises improve physical strength and promote a sense of accomplishment and confidence.
- Yoga combines physical postures with breathwork and meditation, making it an excellent practice for reducing stress and improving mental clarity. Regular yoga practice can help balance the nervous system and promote overall well-being.
- **Tai Chi**: This ancient Chinese practice involves slow, controlled movements and deep breathing. Tai Chi is known to reduce stress, improve balance, and enhance mental clarity.

1. Recognizing Signs of Mental Health Issues

Recognizing the early signs of mental health issues is crucial for seeking timely help and support. Mental health problems often manifest in various ways, both emotionally and physically. Identifying these signs can help individuals take proactive steps to manage their mental well-being.

3.1. Emotional and Behavioral Signs

- **Persistent Sadness or Irritability**: Feeling sad or irritable for long periods without any apparent reason may indicate depression or another mental health issue. This emotional state can affect daily functioning and relationships.
- **Excessive Worry or Fear**: Constantly feeling anxious, fearful, or worried about situations that typically wouldn't cause stress may be a sign of anxiety disorders. This can lead to avoidance behavior and a decreased quality of life.
- **Mood Swings**: Extreme mood swings or fluctuations in behavior may indicate conditions such as bipolar disorder or borderline personality disorder. These mood changes can be rapid and intense, often interfering with daily life.
- **Social Withdrawal**: Isolating oneself from friends, family, or activities that were once enjoyable is a common sign of depression or other mental health conditions. Social withdrawal can exacerbate feelings of loneliness and helplessness.

3.2. Physical Signs

- **Fatigue and Low Energy**: Persistent fatigue, even after adequate rest, can be a sign of depression, anxiety, or other

Chapter 5: Heart Health: The Silent Threat

Introduction to Heart Health and Men's Vulnerability

Heart disease is one of the leading causes of death worldwide, and men are particularly vulnerable to its effects. Often referred to as the "silent killer," heart disease can develop slowly without symptoms, making it difficult to detect until it's too late. Understanding the importance of heart health and taking proactive measures can prevent many associated conditions.

In this chapter, we will explore the most common heart diseases affecting men, identify the risk factors contributing to these diseases, and discuss lifestyle changes and preventive measures to improve heart health.

1. **Common Heart Diseases Affecting Men**

1.1 coronary artery disease (CAD)

Coronary Artery Disease is one of the most common and dangerous heart diseases. It is characterized by the buildup of plaque inside the coronary arteries. The plaque, made up of fatty deposits, cholesterol, and other substances, narrows the arteries, restricting blood flow to the heart. This can lead to chest pain (angina), heart attacks, and even heart failure.

- **Symptoms**: Chest pain, shortness of breath, fatigue, dizziness, and irregular heartbeat.
- **Causes**: High cholesterol, high blood pressure, smoking, diabetes, and a sedentary lifestyle.

1.2 Heart Attack (Myocardial Infarction)

A heart attack occurs when the blood flow to a part of the heart muscle is blocked, leading to tissue damage. This blockage is usually caused by a blood clot forming on a ruptured plaque in the arteries.

- **Symptoms**: Sudden chest pain or discomfort, pain in the arms, neck, or jaw, shortness of breath, and cold sweats.
- **Causes**: Blocked coronary arteries, high cholesterol, hypertension, and smoking.

1.3 Heart Failure

Heart failure is a chronic condition in which the heart cannot pump blood effectively, leading to decreased oxygen supply to the body. It can develop due to coronary artery disease, heart attacks, or high blood pressure.

- **Symptoms** include shortness of breath, fatigue, fluid retention (swelling), rapid heartbeat, and difficulty performing physical activities.
- **Causes**: Previous heart attacks, uncontrolled hypertension, and poor lifestyle choices.

1.4 Arrhythmias

Arrhythmias are abnormal heart rhythms that can lead to heart attacks or strokes. The most common type of arrhythmia is atrial fibrillation (AF), which is characterized by an irregular and often rapid heartbeat. This condition increases the risk of blood clots and can lead to stroke.

- **Symptoms**: Palpitations, dizziness, fatigue, chest pain, and fainting.
- **Causes**: Heart disease, high blood pressure, alcohol consumption, and drug use.

1.5 High Blood Pressure (Hypertension)

Hypertension is one of the most prevalent risk factors for cardiovascular disease. It refers to consistently elevated blood pressure, which can cause damage to the arteries over time. This increases the risk of heart disease, stroke, and kidney failure.

- **Symptoms**: Often known as the "silent killer," hypertension usually doesn't have any symptoms until it's advanced. Some people may experience headaches, dizziness, or shortness of breath.
- **Causes**: Poor diet, lack of physical activity, obesity, excessive alcohol consumption, and genetic factors.

1.6 Aortic Aneurysm

An aortic aneurysm occurs when a section of the aorta (the large artery that carries blood from the heart to the rest of the body) weakens and bulges. If it ruptures, it can be life-threatening.

- **Symptoms**: Severe pain in the chest or abdomen, shortness of breath, and fainting.
- **Causes**: High blood pressure, smoking, and genetic conditions.

1. **Risk Factors for Heart Disease**

While some risk factors for heart disease cannot be changed (such as genetics and age), many can be controlled through lifestyle changes and medical interventions.

2.1 Uncontrollable Risk Factors

- **Age**: The risk of heart disease increases with age. Men over 45 are at higher risk, as the heart and arteries weaken over time.
- **Gender**: Men are generally at a higher risk for heart disease than women, particularly before the age of 55. However, the risk for women increases after menopause.
- **Family History**: A family history of heart disease increases the likelihood of developing heart conditions, mainly if close relatives (parents or siblings) were diagnosed at an early age.

2.2 Controllable Risk Factors

- **High Blood Pressure (Hypertension)**: Elevated blood pressure strains the heart and arteries, making them more likely to develop plaque buildup.
- **High Cholesterol**: Elevated LDL (bad) cholesterol levels can contribute to plaque buildup in the arteries, increasing the risk of CAD and heart attacks.

- **Diabetes**: People with diabetes are at a higher risk of developing heart disease. High blood sugar levels can damage blood vessels over time, increasing the risk of atherosclerosis (narrowing of the arteries).
- **Obesity**: Being overweight or obese contributes to various heart disease risk factors, including hypertension, high cholesterol, and diabetes.
- **Smoking**: Tobacco smoke contains harmful chemicals that damage the blood vessels and promote plaque buildup, which can lead to CAD and heart attacks.
- **Physical Inactivity**: Lack of exercise leads to obesity, high blood pressure, and high cholesterol, all of which increase the risk of heart disease.
- **Excessive Alcohol Consumption**: Drinking too much alcohol can raise blood pressure, lead to irregular heart rhythms, and contribute to weight gain.

1. **Preventive Measures for Heart Disease**

Preventing heart disease is much easier and more effective than treating it once it develops. A proactive approach involves reducing risk factors and adopting heart-healthy habits.

3.1 Regular Check-ups and Screenings

Regular medical check-ups are essential for identifying risk factors early. These check-ups should include monitoring blood pressure, cholesterol levels, and blood sugar. Early detection can help manage risk factors effectively and reduce the likelihood of developing heart disease.

3.2 Medications for Managing Risk Factors

For individuals with high blood pressure, high cholesterol, or diabetes, medications may be prescribed to manage these conditions and reduce the risk of heart disease. Common medications include:

- **Statins**: Used to lower LDL cholesterol.
- **Beta-blockers**: Used to reduce blood pressure and prevent heart attacks.
- **Antiplatelet drugs** Help prevent blood clots, especially in individuals with CAD.
- **Angiotensin-converting enzyme (ACE) inhibitors** Help control blood pressure and protect the heart.

3.3 Controlling Blood Pressure

Managing high blood pressure through lifestyle changes and medications is crucial for heart disease prevention. Reducing sodium intake, increasing potassium-rich foods, managing stress, and regular physical activity can help keep blood pressure in check.

3.4 Controlling Cholesterol Levels

Maintaining healthy cholesterol levels is essential for preventing heart disease. A diet low in saturated and trans fats, regular exercise, and medications (if necessary) can help lower LDL cholesterol and increase HDL (good) cholesterol.

3.5 Diabetes Management

Controlling blood sugar levels is vital in preventing heart disease for individuals with diabetes. A healthy diet, regular exercise, weight management, and medication (e.g., insulin or oral) can help manage blood sugar levels effectively.

1. **Lifestyle Changes to Improve Heart Health**

4.1 Dietary Modifications

A heart-healthy diet plays a significant role in preventing and managing heart disease. Focus on eating nutrient-rich, low-fat foods:

- **Increase Fiber Intake**: Consume more fruits, vegetables, whole grains, and legumes to boost fiber intake, which can help reduce cholesterol and improve heart health.
- **Limit Saturated and Trans Fats**: Avoid foods rich in unhealthy fats, such as fried foods, processed snacks, and fatty cuts of meat. opt for healthy fats like olive oil, nuts, and avocados.
- **Reduce Sodium Intake**: Excessive salt can raise blood pressure. Choose fresh, unprocessed foods and limit high-sodium foods such as canned soups, processed meats, and salty snacks.
- **Increase Omega-3 Fatty Acids**: Omega-3s found in fatty fishlike salmon, mackerel, and sardines can reduce inflammation and lower the risk of heart disease.

4.2 Exercise and Physical Activity

Regular physical activity strengthens the heart, improves circulation, and helps manage weight. Aim for at least 150 minutes of moderate aerobic exercise per week, such as brisk walking or cycling. Resistance training, such as weight lifting, can also improve cardiovascular health by building muscle and increasing metabolism.

4.3 Weight Management

Maintaining a healthy weight reduces the strain on the heart and helps manage other risk factors, such as high blood pressure and diabetes. The best approach to achieving and maintaining a healthy weight is a combination of a healthy diet and regular exercise.

4.4 Stress Management

Chronic stress is a significant contributor to heart disease. Stress can lead to unhealthy habits like overeating, smoking, and excessive drinking. Relaxing techniques such as deep breathing, meditation, yoga, or mindfulness can help reduce stress.

Chapter 6: Weight Management Strategies

1. Understanding Obesity and Its Health Implications

Obesity Defined: Obesity is a complex condition characterized by excessive body fat accumulation that presents a health risk. It is usually measured by the body mass index (BMI), which calculates weight relative to height. A BMI of 30 or above is classified as obese. Various factors, including genetics, behavior, environment, and socioeconomic status, can cause obesity.

Causes of Obesity:

- **Genetic Factors**: Genetics play a significant role in an individual's susceptibility to obesity. Some people may inherit genes that influence how their body stores fat, how efficiently they burn calories, or how their appetite is regulated.
- **Behavioral Factors**: Unhealthy eating habits, a sedentary lifestyle, and a lack of physical activity contribute to obesity. The modern environment exacerbates these behavioral factors with the high availability of processed foods, large portion sizes, and sedentary activities (e.g., television watching and desk jobs).
- **Environmental Influences**: Living in an environment that promotes easy access to unhealthy food options, limited access to safe areas for physical activity, and a lack of education about healthy lifestyles can increase the risk of obesity.
- **Psychological Factors**: Stress, emotional eating, and depression are common contributors to overeating. The relationship between emotions and eating behavior can lead to weight gain, which in turn exacerbates mental health challenges, creating a vicious cycle.

Health Implications of Obesity: Obesity has far-reaching physical and mental health effects. It increases the risk for a range of chronic diseases and conditions, such as:

- **Cardiovascular Diseases**: Obesity is a significant risk factor for heart disease, including hypertension (high blood pressure), coronary artery disease, stroke, and heart failure.
- **Type 2 Diabetes**: Excess fat can lead to insulin resistance, making the body less efficient at regulating blood sugar levels. This is one of the most common complications associated with obesity.
- **Sleep Apnea**: Obesity increases the likelihood of obstructive sleep apnea, where breathing stops intermittently during sleep.
- **Joint Problems**: Carrying excess weight strains joints, particularly the knees, hips, and lower back, increasing the risk of osteoarthritis.
- **Mental Health Issues**: People with obesity may suffer from depression, anxiety, and low self-esteem. Social stigma and discrimination can also contribute to mental health challenges.

- **Cancer**: Obesity is linked to several types of cancer, including breast, colon, and liver cancers, due to the increased production of certain hormones and inflammatory substances associated with excess fat.

1. **Effective Weight Loss Strategies: Diet and Exercise**

Role of Diet in Weight Loss: Diet is one of the most critical factors in achieving and maintaining a healthy weight. The following dietary strategies can help promote weight loss:

- **Calorie Deficit**: The basic principle of weight loss is to consume fewer calories than the body burns. A calorie deficit can be achieved through dietary changes, exercise, or both.
- **Balanced Macronutrients**: A healthy diet should provide an appropriate balance of macronutrients—carbohydrates, proteins, and fats. Each macronutrient serves a different function in the body, and proper intake can help control hunger, maintain muscle mass, and improve metabolic health.
    - **Carbohydrates**: opt for complex carbohydrates (e.g., whole grains, vegetables, legumes) over simple sugars and refined carbs. These foods are more nutrient-dense and promote satiety.
    - **Proteins**: Protein helps preserve muscle mass during weight loss and promotes feelings of fullness. Lean protein sources include chicken, fish, legumes, tofu, and low-fat dairy.
    - **Healthy Fats**: Healthy fats, found in foods like avocados, nuts, seeds, and olive oil, provide essential nutrients and help regulate hormones associated with hunger and metabolism.
- **Portion Control**: Portion control is crucial for reducing calorie intake. Many people underestimate portion sizes, leading to overeating. Using smaller plates, measuring food, and being mindful of portion sizes can help.
- **Meal Timing and Frequency**: Eating smaller, balanced meals throughout the day can help regulate hunger and prevent overeating. Intermittent fasting, though it may only suit some, is successful.
- **Mindful Eating**: Paying attention to hunger cues and eating slowly can help prevent overeating. Mindful eating practices encourage individuals to be more aware of their food choices and portion sizes.

Exercise and Physical Activity: Physical activity is essential for weight management, as it burns calories and improves metabolism and overall health. The main types of exercise for weight loss include:

- **Cardiovascular Exercise (Aerobic Exercise)**: Walking, running, cycling, swimming, and dancing help burn calories and improve heart health. Aim for at least 150 minutes of moderate-intensity aerobic exercise per week.

- **Strength Training (Resistance Exercise)**: Lifting weights, bodyweight exercises, or resistance band workouts build muscle mass, which helps increase metabolic rate and promotes fat loss. Strength training should be done 2-3 times per week.
- **High-Intensity Interval Training (HIIT)**: HIIT involves short bursts of intense activity followed by rest periods or low-intensity exercise. It has been shown to burn more calories quickly and may be particularly effective for fat loss.
- **Flexibility and Mobility Exercises**: Yoga, Pilates, and stretching exercises enhance flexibility and reduce the risk of injury. They are essential for overall fitness and recovery from strength training.

Combining Diet and Exercise for Optimal Results: The most effective weight loss strategies combine diet and exercise. Exercise alone may not lead to significant weight loss without a healthy diet, as people may overcompensate by eating more. Similarly, while diet is critical, regular exercise helps preserve lean muscle mass and improve metabolic rate. A combined approach can also improve overall physical and mental well-being.

1. **Setting Realistic Goals and Tracking Progress**

Setting Realistic Weight Loss Goals: Setting achievable and realistic goals is crucial for long-term success. Unrealistic goals can lead to frustration, burnout, and eventual weight regain. Here are some tips for setting practical goals:

- **SMART Goals**: Goals should be Specific, Measurable, Achievable, Relevant, and Time-bound. For example, instead of saying, "I want to lose weight," a SMART goal would be, "I will lose 1-2 pounds per week for the next 12 weeks."
- **Focus on Non-Scale Victories**: While the scale is an essential tool, it doesn't capture all the health benefits of weight loss. Focus on other progress markers, such as improved energy levels, better sleep, increased physical strength, or improved mood.
- **Set Short, and Long-Term Goals**: Long-term goals (e.g., losing 30 pounds in six months) should be broken down into smaller, short-term goals (e.g., losing 1-2 pounds per week). This approach helps maintain motivation and track progress.
- **Adjust Goals as Needed**: Weight loss is not always linear, and it's essential to remain flexible. If progress stalls or setbacks occur, adjust goals as necessary rather than abandoning them altogether.

Tracking Progress: Tracking progress is essential for staying on track and adjusting your strategies when needed. Several methods can be used to monitor progress:

- **Weighing Yourself**: Weighing yourself regularly (e.g., once a week) can provide insight into overall progress. However, fluctuations are expected, and weight may not reflect changes in body composition.
- **Body Measurements**: Measuring the waist, hips, arms, and legs can provide more insight into body composition changes. Sometimes, fat loss occurs even if the scale doesn't move significantly.
- **Fitness Progress**: Tracking strength, stamina, and endurance improvements can help you assess how well your exercise regimen works. For example, lifting heavier weights, running longer distances, or completing more repetitions indicates progress.
- **Food Journals**: Writing down what you eat helps increase awareness of your eating habits. It can reveal patterns and areas that need improvement, making it easier to make healthier choices.

Dealing with Plateaus and Setbacks: Weight loss plateaus are common and can occur for various reasons, such as hormonal changes, decreased metabolic rate, or muscle gain. When plateaus happen, it's important not to get discouraged. Adjust your diet, exercise routine, or goals to break the plateau. Remember, weight management is a long-term journey, and persistence is key.

Building Support Systems: A support system can significantly enhance weight loss success. This could include family, friends, or a professional such as a dietitian or personal trainer. Social support can help with accountability, motivation, and emotional encouragement during the challenging times of weight management.

Chapter 7: The Importance of Sleep

Introduction to Sleep, Sleep is a vital physiological process for maintaining physical and mental health. It is a complex, restorative activity that allows the body to repair, regenerate, and rejuvenate itself, contributing to emotional well-being and cognitive performance. Yet, despite its importance, sleep is often neglected in modern society due to the demands of work, social life, and various environmental factors. Understanding the role of sleep in overall health, recognizing sleep disorders, and learning tips for improving sleep quality are essential to leading a healthier life.

1. The Role of Sleep in Overall Health

1.1 Sleep as a Restorative Process Sleep is a critical period of bodily repair and maintenance. During sleep, the body's cells regenerate, muscle tissues heal, and the immune system strengthens. Research has demonstrated that adequate sleep is linked to the production of growth hormones, which are essential for cell repair and regeneration. For example, deep sleep (slow-wave sleep) plays a significant role in tissue growth and muscle repair.

Furthermore, sleep is crucial for brain health. It helps clear the brain of toxins accumulated during wakefulness, particularly a protein called beta-amyloid, associated with Alzheimer's disease. Sleep also facilitates memory consolidation and cognitive function, strengthening the connections formed throughout the day and promoting learning.

1.2 Sleep and Physical Health Adequate sleep has direct effects on physical health. Sleep deeply influences the body's metabolic processes, particularly energy regulation and weight control. Chronic sleep deprivation has been linked to increased risk factors for obesity and metabolic syndrome, as it can disrupt hormonal balance. Specifically, sleep deprivation can elevate levels of ghrelin (the hunger hormone) while suppressing leptin (the hormone that signals satiety), leading to overeating and weight gain.

In addition, sleep is vital for cardiovascular health. During sleep, the heart rate and blood pressure drop, which gives the cardiovascular system a chance to rest. Chronic sleep deprivation has been linked to an increased risk of hypertension, heart disease, and stroke.

1.3 Sleep and Mental Health The relationship between sleep and mental health is bidirectional. Poor sleep can exacerbate mental health conditions such as depression, anxiety, and stress, while mental health disorders can lead to sleep disturbances. Sleep is essential for emotional regulation, and insufficient sleep can impair one's ability to manage stress and emotions effectively. Additionally, research shows that lack of sleep increases activity in brain areas responsible for emotional reactivity, making individuals more prone to negative feelings.

Sleep also regulates cortisol levels, which support the body's stress response. Elevated cortisol levels, common during periods of inadequate sleep, can increase inflammation, weaken the immune system, and negatively affect brain function.

1.4 Sleep and Longevity The importance of sleep extends to overall life expectancy. Studies have shown that individuals who consistently get 7 to 9 hours of sleep per night tend to live longer than those who get too little or too much sleep. Insufficient sleep has been linked to a variety of chronic conditions, such as diabetes, hypertension, and obesity, all of which can reduce life expectancy.

A well-balanced sleep schedule contributes to the body's circadian rhythm, which regulates various bodily functions such as hormone release, metabolism, and the immune system. Proper sleep helps maintain the body's natural rhythm, improving overall longevity.

1. Common Sleep Disorders in Men

2.1 Insomnia, Insomnia, is one of the most common sleep disorders, affecting millions worldwide. It is characterized by difficulty falling asleep, staying asleep, or waking up too early. While insomnia can occur in both men and women, it tends to affect men more frequently due to stress and lifestyle factors.

Men with insomnia often experience daytime fatigue, irritability, and difficulty concentrating, which can impact their personal and professional lives. Chronic insomnia can increase the risk of developing other health problems, such as depression, anxiety, and cardiovascular diseases.

2.2 Sleep Apnea Sleep apnea, particularly obstructive sleep apnea (OSA), is a sleep disorder in which breathing repeatedly stops and starts during sleep. This disorder is particularly prevalent among men, especially those who are overweight or have a family history of sleep apnea.

Sleep apnea can cause loud snoring, choking, gasping during sleep, and excessive daytime sleepiness in men. Left untreated, sleep apnea increases the risk of heart disease, stroke, and high blood pressure. It can also lead to cognitive problems, mood disorders, and a reduced quality of life.

2.3 Restless Legs Syndrome (RLS) is characterized by an uncontrollable urge to move the legs, particularly when at rest or trying to sleep. Men with RLS often report a sensation of crawling, tingling, or itching in their legs, which can interfere with their ability to fall asleep or stay asleep. The discomfort typically worsens during periods of inactivity and improves with movement.

RLS is more common in middle-aged and older men, and it has been linked to other conditions such as iron deficiency, kidney disease, and diabetes. Although RLS can affect women as well, it tends to be more pronounced in men.

2.4 Narcolepsy, Narcolepsy, is a neurological condition that causes excessive daytime sleepiness and sudden sleep attacks. Men are more likely than women to experience severe symptoms of narcolepsy, which include episodes of sudden, uncontrollable sleep during the day, regardless of activity. Narcolepsy is often accompanied by cataplexy, a sudden loss of muscle strength triggered by emotions such as laughter or surprise.

Although the condition is rare, narcolepsy can significantly impair a person's quality of life, as it often leads to difficulties with work, relationships, and general daily functioning. The exact cause of narcolepsy remains unclear, but it is believed to be related to genetic and autoimmune factors.

2.5 Circadian Rhythm Disorders Men, especially those with demanding work schedules, may develop circadian rhythm disorders. These disorders occur when the body's internal clock becomes misaligned with the external environment. Shift work, jet lag, and irregular sleep schedules can disrupt the natural rhythm of sleep-wake cycles, leading to problems falling asleep, staying asleep, and experiencing restorative sleep.

Circadian rhythm disorders are common among men who work night shifts or travel frequently across time zones. These disorders can result in chronic fatigue, poor concentration, irritability, and even depression.

1. Tips for Improving Sleep Quality

3.1 Establishing a Consistent Sleep Schedule One of the most effective ways to improve sleep quality is to establish a regular sleep schedule. Going to bed and waking up simultaneously daily, including on weekends, helps regulate the body's circadian rhythm. This consistency improves the likelihood of falling asleep and waking up feeling refreshed.

Men with irregular sleep patterns, such as those who work shifts or experience jet lag, should try to gradually adjust their sleep times to align with their natural sleep-wake cycle.

3.2 Creating a Sleep-Friendly Environment The environment in which one sleeps plays a crucial role in sleep quality. Men should create a calm, quiet environment to encourage better sleep. The ideal room temperature for sleep is typically between 60-67°F (15-19°C), as it supports the body's natural drop in temperature during sleep.

Eliminating noise and light can also enhance sleep quality. Blackout curtains, earplugs, or a white noise machine can help minimize disturbances. Furthermore, a comfortable mattress and pillows are essential for promoting restful sleep.

3.3 Managing Stress and Anxiety Stress and anxiety are significant barriers to good sleep. Men who find it difficult to fall asleep due to racing thoughts or worrying about daily responsibilities should consider stress-reduction techniques such as mindfulness meditation, deep breathing exercises, or progressive muscle relaxation.

Journaling before bed can also help reduce stress by allowing men to express their thoughts and clear their minds. Physical exercise is another proven method for alleviating stress and promoting better sleep. However, avoiding vigorous exercise close to bedtime is essential, as it may have an energizing effect.

3.4 Limiting Caffeine and Alcohol Intake Caffeine and alcohol can disrupt sleep if consumed too late in the day. Caffeine, found in coffee, tea, and certain sodas, is a stimulant that can interfere with the ability to fall asleep. Limiting caffeine consumption to the morning and early afternoon hours is advisable.

Similarly, while alcohol may make individuals feel drowsy initially, it can disrupt sleep during the night, particularly in the second half of the sleep cycle. Limiting alcohol intake, incredibly close to bedtime, can lead to more restful sleep.

3.5 Exercise and Physical Activity Regular physical activity can significantly improve sleep quality. Exercise helps regulate the body's internal clock, promoting more profound and more restful sleep. It also reduces insomnia and sleep apnea symptoms by improving overall cardiovascular health.

However, timing is essential when it comes to exercise. Strenuous exercise close to bedtime can have the opposite effect, increasing energy levels and making it harder to fall asleep. Ideally, training should be completed a few hours before bedtime.

3.6 Nutrition and Sleep Dietary choices can also affect sleep quality. Eating heavy or spicy meals before bed can lead to indigestion or heartburn, making sleeping difficult. Men should aim to have their last meal at least 2-3 hours before bedtime and focus on light, nutritious foods that support sleep.

Certain foods, such as those rich in tryptophan (e.g., turkey, nuts, and seeds), magnesium, and melatonin,

Chapter 8: Preventive Care and Regular Check-Ups

Preventive care and regular check-ups are crucial to maintaining optimal health throughout life. In a world where medical conditions often develop gradually and may not show symptoms until they become severe, proactive health management is essential. This chapter explores the significance of preventive care, outlines recommended tests and screenings, and emphasizes the importance of building a strong relationship with healthcare providers for long-term health benefits.

8.1 Importance of Regular Health Screenings

Health screenings are one of the most effective ways to detect and prevent potential health problems before they become more severe. The key idea behind preventive healthcare is to identify risk factors early, address them in their early stages, and prevent the onset of chronic diseases, thereby improving overall quality of life.

8.1.1 Early Detection of Diseases

Many diseases, such as heart disease, diabetes, and certain cancers, can be managed or even cured more effectively when detected early. Health screenings provide valuable insights into a person's current health status, helping to identify risk factors or early signs of conditions that could otherwise go unnoticed. For instance, high blood pressure often has no symptoms but, left unchecked, it can lead to severe complications like stroke or kidney failure. Regular screenings ensure that such silent conditions are identified before they escalate.

8.1.2 Preventing Chronic Illnesses

Preventive care aims to catch potential health problems in their infancy. By addressing these issues early, individuals can avoid developing chronic, lifelong conditions that could otherwise require intensive medical treatment. For example, lifestyle changes prompted by screening results for high cholesterol or diabetes can prevent or delay the onset of cardiovascular diseases or other complications. This improves the quality of life and reduces long-term healthcare costs associated with treating advanced conditions.

8.1.3 Health Promotion and Education

Preventive care is also a platform for educating individuals about their health and the steps they can take to live healthier lives. Screenings and check-ups allow one to discuss diet, exercise, mental health, and lifestyle habits contributing to potential health risks. These check-ups are often the first step in encouraging individuals to engage in healthy behaviors that prevent future health problems.

8.1.4 Mental Health Monitoring

Mental health conditions, such as anxiety, depression, and stress, can have significant physical consequences if left unaddressed. Regular check-ups offer a chance to assess not only physical health but also mental well-being.

Screening tools, questionnaires, and discussions about stress levels, sleep patterns, and emotional health can help healthcare providers spot early signs of mental health issues and provide appropriate interventions.

8.2 Recommended Tests and Their Frequency

The tests you need will depend on your age, gender, health history, and lifestyle. Regular screening can catch health issues early, but it is equally important to know which tests are essential and how often to get them. Below is a breakdown of standard health screenings and tests for adults, categorized by age and gender.

8.2.1 Blood Pressure Screening

Blood pressure is one of the simplest and most effective ways to assess cardiovascular health. High blood pressure is known as the "silent killer" because it often has no noticeable symptoms but can cause damage to the heart, kidneys, and arteries.

- **Frequency**: Adults should check their blood pressure at least once every two years or more if they are at risk of high blood pressure.
- **Recommended Age**: Starting at age 18 for adults, with increased frequency after age 40 or if there are risk factors such as obesity or a family history of hypertension.

8.2.2 Cholesterol Levels and Lipid Profile

A cholesterol test, also known as a lipid profile, measures the levels of various types of fat in your blood. High cholesterol is a significant risk factor for heart disease and stroke.

- **Frequency**: Adults should have their cholesterol checked every 4-6 years. People at higher risk (those with a family history of heart disease, diabetes, or high blood pressure) may need more frequent screenings.
- **Recommended Age**: Starting at age 20, with increased frequency after age 40 or if you are at increased risk of heart disease.

8.2.3 Blood Sugar Test

Testing for blood sugar is essential in detecting diabetes, a disease that affects millions of people worldwide. Early diagnosis can lead to better management of the condition and prevent complications.

- **Frequency**: Adults should be tested every three years for diabetes, starting at age 45 or earlier, for those with risk factors (obesity, sedentary lifestyle, or family history).
- **Recommended Age**: Starting at age 45 or earlier if risk factors exist.

8.2.4 Cancer Screenings

Regular cancer screenings are critical for detecting certain types of cancer early. The specific types of cancer that must be screened for vary by gender and risk factors.

- **Breast Cancer**: Mammograms are recommended for women starting at age 40 and continuing every 1-2 years.

- **Cervical Cancer**: Pap smears and HPV tests are recommended for women beginning at age 21, every 3 years until age 29, and then every 5 years until age 65.
- **Prostate Cancer**: For men, prostate exams and PSA (Prostate-Specific Antigen) testing may begin at age 50 or earlier if there are risk factors like family history.
- **Colorectal Cancer**: Colonoscopy is recommended for both men and women at age 45 and every 10 years after that or earlier if risk factors exist (e.g., family history of colorectal cancer).

8.2.5 Bone Density Test

A bone density test can detect osteoporosis, which weakens bones and increases the risk of fractures.

- **Frequency**: Typically, a bone density test is recommended once for women over 65 and men over 70 or earlier if there are risk factors such as a family history of osteoporosis, smoking, or a sedentary lifestyle.

8.2.6 Vision and Hearing Tests

Vision and hearing tests are essential in identifying early issues related to sight and hearing that could affect quality of life.

- **Frequency**: Adults should have vision exams every 2 years and hearing tests at least once every decade until age 50 and every 3 years after that.

8.2.7 Skin Cancer Screening

Skin cancer is one of the most common types of cancer, and early detection is critical for effective treatment. A full-body skin examination is recommended to identify any unusual moles or skin changes.

- **Frequency**: A skin check should be done yearly, especially for people with a family history of skin cancer or those who spend a lot of time in the sun.

8.2.8 Vaccinations

While vaccinations are typically associated with children, adults must stay updated with their immunizations.

- **Recommended Vaccines**: Influenza, pneumonia, hepatitis B, and shingles vaccines are typically recommended for older adults or those with chronic illnesses.
- **Frequency**: Vaccines should be administered as per public health guidelines, often on a yearly or decadal basis.

8.3 Building a Relationship with Healthcare Providers

A strong relationship with a healthcare provider is the cornerstone of effective preventive care. This relationship is built on trust, communication, and mutual respect, empowering individuals to manage their health actively.

8.3.1 Continuity of Care

Seeing the same healthcare provider over time allows for continuity of care. Your doctor is familiar with your health history, concerns, and lifestyle, which helps your provider make personalized recommendations, track progress, and catch potential health problems early.

- **Importance of Consistency**: Regular visits to the same provider help ensure that they are up to date with your medical history and any conditions you may have.
- **Building Trust**: Establishing trust with your healthcare provider ensures that you feel comfortable discussing sensitive issues, such as mental health, sexual health, or substance abuse, which could impact your overall health.

8.3.2 Open Communication

Effective communication is key to any successful doctor-patient relationship. Being honest and transparent with your healthcare provider about your symptoms, lifestyle habits, and concerns is essential. This helps the provider make informed decisions about your care and can lead to better outcomes.

- **Asking Questions**: Don't hesitate to ask your healthcare provider questions if you don't understand a diagnosis, treatment, or preventive measure.
- **Sharing Lifestyle Information**: Be open about your diet, exercise, stress levels, and any other factors that may affect your health.

8.3.3 Advocating for Yourself

Building a relationship with your healthcare provider also involves advocating for your health. This means being an active participant in decisions regarding your health and well-being.

- **Seeking Second Opinions**: If you are ever uncertain about a diagnosis or treatment plan, seeking a second opinion is essential to ensure you get the best possible care.
- **Knowing Your Rights**: Be aware of your rights as a patient, including your right to access your medical records, ask for explanations of procedures, and make informed decisions about your care.

Conclusion

Preventive care and regular check-ups are fundamental to maintaining a long and healthy life. By prioritizing regular screenings, understanding the tests necessary for early detection, and fostering strong relationships with healthcare providers, individuals can

Chapter 9: Sexual Health and Wellness

Sexual health is integral to overall well-being, and understanding its nuances is critical for maintaining a healthy relationship with oneself and others. This chapter will explore common sexual health issues faced by men, the importance of open communication with partners, and the resources available for sexual health education. It aims to offer insight into the complex nature of sexual health and how individuals can cultivate a fulfilling, respectful, and informed sexual life.

1. **Common Sexual Health Issues Faced by Men**

Men, like women, face a variety of sexual health issues that can range from physiological concerns to emotional and psychological challenges. These issues can impact self-esteem, relationship satisfaction, and overall health. Addressing them openly can improve both sexual health and emotional well-being.

1.1 Erectile Dysfunction (ED)

Erectile dysfunction, or impotence, is one of the most commonly discussed sexual health issues among men. It refers to the inability to achieve or maintain an erection firm enough for sexual intercourse. ED can result from a variety of factors, including:

- **Physical Causes**: Conditions such as diabetes, heart disease, high blood pressure, obesity, and hormonal imbalances are among the leading physical causes of ED. The narrowing of blood vessels, mainly due to atherosclerosis (hardening of the arteries), can affect blood flow to the penis, making it difficult to achieve an erection.
- **Psychological Causes**: Stress, anxiety, depression, and relationship problems can also contribute to ED. Performance anxiety, fear of rejection, or unresolved emotional issues can significantly impact sexual performance.
- **Medications**: Certain medications, including antidepressants, antihypertensives, and tranquilizers, can interfere with sexual function. Therefore, men experiencing ED must review their medication lists with healthcare providers.
- **Age**: While ED is more common as men age, it is not inevitable. Lifestyle changes, such as improved diet and exercise, can help mitigate its effects.

1.2 Premature Ejaculation

Premature ejaculation (PE) is when a man ejaculates too quickly during sexual intercourse, often before either partner is satisfied. This issue can be highly distressing and impact relationship dynamics. Several factors may cause it:

- **Psychological Factors**: Anxiety, stress, and performance pressure can lead to rapid ejaculation. Often, these psychological triggers may be linked to a man's early sexual experiences.
- **Medical Conditions**: Hormonal imbalances, infections, or prostatitis (prostate inflammation) can contribute to PE. Neurological issues and thyroid problems may also play a role.
- **Behavioral Causes**: Lack of sexual experience or rushing through intercourse can lead to premature ejaculation. Men who have not had the opportunity to learn to control their arousal levels may experience difficulty.

Treatment for PE often involves therapy (behavioral or cognitive), medications, or lifestyle changes to reduce anxiety and improve sexual function.

1.3 Low Libido and Sexual Desire

A decrease in sexual desire or libido is another common issue among men, often related to a range of factors:

- **Hormonal Imbalances**: Testosterone, the hormone responsible for regulating sexual desire, may decline due to aging, stress, or medical conditions like hypogonadism. Low testosterone levels can lead to reduced libido.
- **Mental Health**: Conditions such as depression, anxiety, or low self-esteem can negatively affect a man's desire for sex. Relationship dissatisfaction, including unresolved conflicts or emotional distance, can also lead to low libido.
- **Lifestyle Factors**: Excessive alcohol consumption, drug use, lack of exercise, and poor diet are lifestyle choices that can hinder sexual desire. Managing these factors is key to maintaining a healthy libido.

Treatments include testosterone therapy, counseling, lifestyle modifications, and sometimes medications that address underlying causes.

1.4 Sexually Transmitted Infections (STIs)

STIs represent a significant sexual health risk and can affect anyone, regardless of gender. Common STIs that impact men include:

- **Chlamydia**: Often asymptomatic, chlamydia can cause pain during urination or discharge from the penis. Untreated, it may lead to complications such as infertility.
- **Gonorrhea**: Like chlamydia, gonorrhea can cause pain during urination and discharge. It may also lead to more serious complications if untreated, including epididymitis and infertility.
- **Herpes Simplex Virus (HSV)**: HSV-1 and HSV-2 can cause painful sores and blisters around the genital area. While there is no cure, antiviral medications can help manage outbreaks.

- **Human Papillomavirus (HPV)**: Certain strains of HPV can cause genital warts, while others are linked to cancers of the penis, anus, and throat.

Regular screening for STIs and using protection (e.g., condoms) during sexual activity are essential preventive measures.

1.5 Low Sperm Count and Infertility

Male infertility, often caused by a low sperm count, can be a distressing issue for couples trying to conceive. Contributing factors include:

- **Varicocele**: Enlarged veins in the scrotum can lead to reduced sperm production and quality.
- **Infections**: Sexually transmitted infections, as well as other diseases of the reproductive organs, can impair sperm production.
- **Lifestyle Choices**: Smoking, excessive alcohol consumption, and exposure to environmental toxins (e.g., pesticides, lead) can negatively affect sperm count.

Treatment may involve lifestyle changes, medications, or assisted reproductive technologies like in-vitro fertilization (IVF).

1. **Importance of Open Communication with Partners**

Communication is the cornerstone of any healthy relationship, particularly regarding sexual health and wellness. Open dialogue allows couples to understand each other's needs, address concerns, and create a safe space for both partners to express their desires and boundaries.

2.1 Building Trust and Comfort

Sexual health issues, such as ED, low libido, or STIs, can often cause embarrassment or anxiety. In such cases, a partner's support is vital. When both partners are open about their sexual needs, concerns, and health status, it fosters a sense of trust and comfort.

- **Emotional Safety**: Men are often socialized to view vulnerability as a weakness, but opening up about sexual difficulties can improve intimacy and connection. Being open reduces the emotional stress associated with sexual health problems.
- **Reassurance**: A partner who is understanding and empathetic can alleviate the anxiety that comes with issues like premature ejaculation

or erectile dysfunction. Communication reassures both partners that they are doing this together.

2.2 Discussing Preferences and Boundaries

Sexual compatibility goes beyond physical attraction; it includes a mutual understanding of preferences, boundaries, and desires. Open communication allows both partners to negotiate their needs and desires, creating a fulfilling and respectful sexual experience.

- **Consent**: An open dialogue ensures that both partners are comfortable with the sexual activity they engage in. Consent should be continuous and communicated freely.
- **Mutual Satisfaction**: Discussing likes, dislikes, and what feels good ensures that both partners are satisfied with their sexual experiences. This also includes discussing the use of contraception, sexual health practices, and any limitations or needs.

2.3 Addressing Health Issues

When one or both partners face sexual health concerns, discussing them openly can help identify solutions and strategies. For example, a man experiencing ED or low libido may feel pressure to perform. Still, a candid conversation allows the couple to address the issue together, whether it be through seeking medical help or exploring other forms of intimacy.

- **Seeking Medical Advice Together**: When one partner faces a sexual health challenge, it is often helpful for both partners to go together to a healthcare provider. This shows support and makes the process feel less isolating.
- **Honesty About STI Risks**: Regular STI testing, especially in new or multiple-partner relationships, ensures that both individuals are protected and can make informed choices about sexual activities.

2.4 Benefits of Open Communication

Open communication contributes not only to sexual health but also to emotional and psychological well-being. It helps:

- **Enhance Emotional Intimacy**: Sharing sexual health concerns can foster deeper emotional intimacy. When both partners feel heard and understood, their bond is strengthened.

- **Improve Physical Health**: By talking about sexual health, couples are more likely to take proactive steps in preventing or addressing issues such as STIs, erectile dysfunction, and low libido.

1. **Resources for Sexual Health Education**

Access to accurate and comprehensive sexual health education is essential for promoting well-being and preventing issues related to sexual health. There are numerous resources available that can provide men with the knowledge they need to take care of their sexual health.

3.1 Healthcare Providers

Primary care physicians, urologists, and sexual health specialists are among the most valuable resources for sexual health. These professionals can:

- Diagnose and treat sexual health conditions like erectile dysfunction, premature ejaculation, or low testosterone.
- Provide counseling on sexual performance anxiety, relationship issues, and mental health.
- Offer STI screenings and vaccinations (e.g., HPV and hepatitis B).

3.2 Online Resources and Websites

Many reputable websites offer information on sexual health topics. These resources can provide valuable advice on various sexual health matters, such as:

- The **American Urological Association** and **American Sexual Health Association** websites offer guidance on issues like erectile dysfunction, fertility, and STIs.
- **Planned Parenthood** offers accessible sexual health information for men and women, addressing everything from contraception to STI prevention.

3.3 Support Groups and Counseling

Support groups provide men with a sense of community when facing sexual health challenges. These groups offer a space for men.

Chapter 10: Building Healthy Relationships

Introduction

Human beings are social creatures, and our connections with others are crucial to our emotional, psychological, and physical well-being. Healthy relationships can lead to increased life satisfaction, improved mental health, and longer life expectancy. In contrast, the absence of meaningful relationships or the presence of toxic ones can harm one's health. This chapter explores the various aspects of building healthy relationships, focusing on the impact of social connections on health, strategies for fostering meaningful relationships, and the importance of support systems.

1. **The Impact of Social Connections on Health**

Our relationships are important for our emotional and psychological happiness, and they also significantly influence our physical health. Several studies have shown that social connections, or the lack thereof, can profoundly affect a person's well-being.

1.1 Social Connections and Longevity

Research has consistently shown that strong social connections can increase life expectancy. A study by the University of California found that people with strong social ties are 50% more likely to live longer than those who are socially isolated. Social interaction has been linked to the regulation of stress hormones, reduction in inflammation, and better immune system function. Individuals with strong social bonds are better able to handle the stresses of life and are less likely to develop chronic illnesses.

1.2 Mental Health and Social Connections

Mental health is closely tied to the quality of one's relationships. People who have strong social support systems tend to experience lower levels of depression, anxiety, and stress. Close friendships and family connections provide a safety net in emotional distress, helping individuals cope with grief, loss, or fear.

For instance, studies have shown that individuals with supportive relationships are less likely to develop anxiety or depression. Social interaction can also act as a protective factor against cognitive decline in older adults. Regular conversations and social activities stimulate the brain and maintain mental health.

1.3 The Physiological Benefits of Healthy Relationships

Healthy relationships can reduce the levels of stress hormones such as cortisol in the body. Chronic stress is known to contribute to a variety of health issues, including heart disease, high blood pressure, and diabetes. The emotional comfort provided by supportive relationships helps buffer the body from the harmful effects of stress.

Research on heart health has also shown that people with strong social networks are less likely to experience heart attacks or strokes. Positive social interactions can improve cardiovascular health by lowering blood pressure and reducing the risk of inflammation, contributing to heart disease.

1.4 Social Isolation and Its Negative Impact on Health

On the opposite end of the spectrum, social isolation can devastate health. Loneliness, which is often associated with social isolation, has been shown to increase the risk of developing various health problems, including cardiovascular disease, stroke, and even early mortality. A study published in PLOS Medicine found that social isolation is as dangerous for health as smoking 15 cigarettes a day.

Loneliness can also lead to poor mental health outcomes, including depression, anxiety, and decreased cognitive function. When people feel disconnected from others, they may struggle to maintain self-care routines, which further exacerbates the risks to their physical health.

1. Strategies for Fostering Meaningful Relationships

Building and maintaining meaningful relationships requires effort, time, and the ability to connect with others on a deeper level. Below are some strategies that can help individuals foster and cultivate healthy, meaningful relationships.

2.1 Practice Active Listening

Active listening is one of the most effective ways to build deeper connections. This involves entirely focusing on what the other person is saying without interrupting or formulating your response while they speak. By actively listening, you demonstrate Empathy and respect, which fosters trust and understanding.

Active listening also means being present at the moment, maintaining eye contact, and using body language to convey attentiveness. These actions help the speaker feel valued and understood, making it easier to form a meaningful connection.

2.2 Open and Honest Communication

Honest communication is a cornerstone of healthy relationships. When people are open and transparent about their thoughts, feelings, and expectations, it builds trust and reduces misunderstandings. Effective communication allows both parties to express their needs, desires, and concerns in a safe and supportive environment.

It is also important to be receptive to feedback. Relationships thrive when individuals are open to constructive criticism and willing to adjust their behavior when necessary. This requires emotional maturity and the ability to manage conflict healthily.

2.3 Cultivate Empathy

Empathy is the ability to understand and share another person's feelings. When we are empathetic, we can better connect with others on an emotional level. Cultivating Empathy involves being attuned to others' emotions, validating their feelings, and offering support when needed.

Empathy is crucial for strengthening relationships and resolving conflicts. By putting ourselves in the other person's shoes, we can approach disagreements with understanding rather than judgment or defensiveness.

2.4 Spend Quality Time Together

In today's fast-paced world, neglecting the importance of spending quality time with loved ones is easy. However, shared experiences help deepen relationships and create lasting bonds. This could involve doing activities together, such as cooking, exercising, or engaging in hobbies. Prioritizing time for these activities is essential, even if it means scheduling them in advance.

Quality time is also about being present and engaged at the moment. Setting aside distractions like phones or work helps foster meaningful interactions and strengthens relationships.

2.5 Show Appreciation and Gratitude

Expressing appreciation and gratitude is a powerful way to reinforce relationships. Through words, actions, or small gestures, showing appreciation helps others feel valued and respected. Simple acts of kindness, such as saying "thank you" or offering support during tough times, go a long way in maintaining positive relationships.

Gratitude can also improve our well-being. Studies have shown that regularly practicing gratitude can increase happiness, reduce stress, and enhance overall mental health.

2.6 Be Vulnerable

Vulnerability is often seen as a weakness, but it is one of the most powerful tools for building meaningful relationships. When we allow ourselves to be vulnerable, we open up to others and invite them to do the same, fostering intimacy and trust.

Being vulnerable can mean sharing our fears, insecurities, or personal challenges. It allows others to see us as human and helps them relate to us deeper. While vulnerability may initially feel uncomfortable, it is essential to create connections built on trust and authenticity.

2.7 Support Others and Ask for Help

Support is a two-way street in any healthy relationship. Offering emotional, physical, or practical support to others helps create a sense of mutual care and understanding. Likewise, it's essential to be open to receiving help when needed. Asking for support is a sign of strength, not weakness, and it strengthens relationships by fostering a sense of interdependence.

When we offer and accept support, we create a dynamic of reciprocity that enhances the bond between individuals.

1. The Role of Support Systems in Health

Support systems are networks of people who provide emotional, social, and practical support. These systems play a vital role in maintaining mental and physical health.

3.1 Types of Support Systems

Support systems can come in many forms, including:

- **Family Support**: Family members are often the first line of support for individuals. They offer emotional support, help with caregiving, and provide financial or practical assistance during difficult times.
- **Friends and Social Networks**: Close friends provide companionship, emotional comfort, and social engagement. Having a wide circle of friends or a strong social network can enhance feelings of belonging and reduce the risks of loneliness.
- **Professional Support**: Healthcare providers, therapists, and counselors must offer professional support. They can help individuals manage mental health issues, chronic illnesses, or personal crises.
- **Community and Peer Support**: Support groups, religious organizations, and community programs offer a sense of connection and belonging. These groups can provide shared experiences, emotional validation, and practical resources.

3.2 Emotional Support

Emotional support is critical for coping with life's challenges. It involves providing comfort, encouragement, and reassurance. Having someone to talk to, especially during times of distress, can help alleviate feelings of loneliness and anxiety.

Emotional support helps individuals manage stress and feel less overwhelmed by difficult situations. This type of support is often the most beneficial in times of emotional crisis, such as during the loss of a loved one, job loss, or personal failure.

3.3 Social Support and Coping Mechanisms

Social support helps individuals cope with challenges in a healthier way. People with strong support systems tend to handle stress better and are less likely to develop harmful coping mechanisms, such as substance abuse or withdrawal. Social support provides an outlet for sharing burdens and seeking guidance.

The presence of supportive people can encourage healthier lifestyle choices, such as regular exercise, eating nutritious meals, and getting adequate sleep. Additionally, social support can motivate individuals to seek medical attention and adhere to treatment plans.

3.4 Physical Support and Assistance

Support systems also provide practical help when needed. This may include assistance with household tasks, transportation, childcare, or caregiving for elderly or ill family members. This type of support is crucial for maintaining physical health and managing daily responsibilities.

Physical support from loved ones or professionals can significantly improve their recovery and well-being when individuals face health challenges.

3.5 The Benefits of Support Systems for Health

The benefits of strong support systems are vast. People with robust support networks experience lower levels of stress, improved immune function, and better overall health outcomes.

Chapter 11: Substance Use and Addiction

1. **Overview of Substance Abuse Issues in Men**

Substance abuse refers to the harmful or hazardous use of psychoactive substances, including alcohol, illicit drugs, and prescription medications, leading to addiction. Addiction, in this context, is characterized by a compulsive need to continue using these substances despite the negative consequences.

1.1 Understanding Substance Use and Addiction in Men

Men are statistically more likely than women to engage in substance use and abuse. Research consistently shows that men tend to start using substances at an earlier age and are more likely to develop substance use disorders (SUDs).

Factors contributing to substance use in men:

- **Biological Factors**: Men have different brain structures and hormonal levels than women, which can influence addiction risks. Higher testosterone levels in men have been linked to impulsive behavior, which can contribute to substance abuse.
- **Psychological Factors**: Men may use substances to cope with mental health issues such as depression, anxiety, or trauma. However, these psychological issues often go unaddressed due to the stigma around mental health among men.
- **Social and Cultural Factors**: Social expectations around masculinity often discourage men from expressing vulnerability or seeking help. As a result, men may use substances as a form of self-medication to manage stress, emotional pain, or difficult life circumstances.
- **Peer Pressure**: Men are more likely than women to be influenced by peers or social circles that normalize heavy drinking, smoking, or drug use. This peer pressure can escalate substance abuse behaviors.
- **Economic and Environmental Stressors**: Men, especially those from lower socioeconomic backgrounds, are more likely to experience stressors such as unemployment, financial instability, or social isolation, all of which are risk factors for substance abuse.

1.2 Patterns of Substance Use in Men

The types of substances most commonly abused by men differ from those abused by women in some key respects:

- **Alcohol Use**: Alcohol consumption is the most widespread form of substance abuse among men. Men are more likely than women to binge drink and develop alcohol dependency. This is often linked to social and cultural practices, where drinking is normalized in many male social circles.

- **Cigarette Smoking**: Smoking rates are generally higher in men, particularly in lower socioeconomic groups. Smoking is often associated with stress management and social gatherings.
- **Illicit Drugs**: Men are more likely to use illegal substances such as marijuana, cocaine, heroin, and methamphetamines. The use patterns vary across different age groups, with younger men being more susceptible to experimentation and risk-taking behaviors.
- **Prescription Drug Misuse**: Men are also more likely to misuse prescription drugs, especially painkillers and stimulants. This is often linked to mental health disorders, physical injuries, or work-related stress.

1.3 The Impact of Substance Abuse on Men's Health

Substance abuse in men can lead to numerous adverse health outcomes, including:

- **Mental Health Disorders**: Men with substance use disorders are more likely to suffer from depression, anxiety, and other mental health conditions, which may exacerbate their substance abuse.
- **Physical Health Complications**: Chronic substance abuse can result in liver disease (due to alcohol), lung disease (due to smoking), cardiovascular problems, and neurological damage.
- **Higher Risk of Violence and Accidents**: Men with substance abuse problems are at a higher risk of engaging in violent behavior or being involved in accidents, including motor vehicle crashes or falls.
- **Family and Relationship Issues**: Substance abuse often causes strain in relationships, leading to domestic violence, neglect, and separation. Children of parents with substance abuse problems are also at higher risk for developing their addiction issues.

1. **Strategies for Prevention and Recovery**

Preventing and recovering from substance use and addiction requires a multifaceted approach that includes education, early intervention, treatment, and ongoing support. The following strategies have been identified as effective in addressing substance abuse among men:

2.1 Prevention of Substance Abuse

Prevention efforts aim to reduce the risk of developing substance use disorders by addressing risk factors before substance use begins.

Key prevention strategies include:

- **Education and Awareness**: Providing information about the risks of substance abuse and promoting healthier coping mechanisms can help individuals, particularly young men, avoid risky behaviors.
- **Promoting Healthy Social Connections**: Encouraging the formation of positive social networks and relationships can act as a protective factor against substance use. Engaging in healthy activities, such as sports, arts, or volunteering, can help men build confidence and emotional resilience.
- **Parent and Family-Based Programs**: Programs targeting families can help parents identify risk factors for substance abuse early and equip them with the tools to talk to their children about substance use.
- **School-Based Programs**: Early education programs in schools can help students understand the risks of substance use and teach them skills to resist peer pressure.
- **Workplace Programs**: Employers can implement workplace wellness programs that educate employees on the dangers of substance abuse and offer support for those struggling with addiction.

2.2 Treatment and Recovery

For men who have developed substance use disorders, treatment and recovery are crucial. There are various treatment models and therapies that can help men manage addiction and work toward long-term recovery.

Key treatment options include:

- **Behavioral Therapy**: Cognitive-behavioral therapy (CBT) is one of the most effective forms of treatment for substance abuse. CBT helps individuals recognize and change unhealthy thought patterns and behaviors associated with substance use.
- **Motivational Interviewing (MI)**: This is a counseling approach that helps individuals explore and resolve ambivalence about their substance use. MI effectively promotes long-term behavior change and motivates individuals to engage in treatment.
- **Residential Treatment Programs**: For men with severe addiction issues, residential treatment may be necessary. These programs provide structured care in a controlled environment and typically offer medical and psychological treatment.
- **Outpatient Treatment Programs**: These programs allow men to receive treatment while continuing to live at home. They may involve

individual therapy, group counseling, and educational sessions on substance use and recovery.

- **Medication-Assisted Treatment (MAT)**: For certain types of addiction, such as opioid or alcohol dependence, MAT can be used to help manage withdrawal symptoms and cravings. Medications like methadone or buprenorphine for opioid addiction and disulfiram or naltrexone for alcohol addiction can help reduce the risk of relapse.
- **Support Groups**: Peer support groups, such as Alcoholics Anonymous (AA) or Narcotics Anonymous (NA), provide a community-based approach to recovery. These groups offer support from others who have faced similar struggles and can share their experiences.

2.3 Building a Recovery-Oriented Lifestyle

For men in recovery, building a lifestyle that supports long-term sobriety is essential. This involves creating a healthy, supportive environment that fosters personal growth and well-being. Strategies include:

- **Creating Healthy Habits**: Men in recovery are encouraged to develop new habits, such as regular exercise, healthy eating, and mindfulness practices, which can improve physical and mental health.
- **Engaging in Meaningful Activities**: Hobbies or new interests can replace the void left by substance use. Many men find fulfillment in sports, creative arts, volunteering, or furthering their education.
- **Establishing Strong Support Networks**: Recovery is often sustained by building supportive relationships with family, friends, and peers who encourage sobriety and provide accountability.

1. **Resources for Seeking Help**

Seeking help is a crucial step for men who are struggling with substance abuse. A variety of resources exist to support men in their journey to recovery.

3.1 Professional Support Services

- **Therapists and Counselors**: Licensed therapists, psychologists, and counselors can provide individual therapy, group counseling, and family therapy. These professionals are trained to help individuals manage addiction and address underlying mental health issues.
- **Treatment Centers and Hospitals**: For individuals needing intensive support, treatment centers provide residential care or outpatient services for detoxification, therapy, and aftercare.

Hospitals can also offer medical detoxification for those who need supervision during the withdrawal process.

- **Substance Abuse Helplines**: Many countries have toll-free helplines for individuals seeking help with substance abuse. These helplines offer confidential support and can provide information on local treatment options.

3.2 Peer Support and Community Resources

- **Support Groups (AA, NA, SMART Recovery)**: Peer support groups are vital for long-term recovery. Organizations like AA and NA offer regular meetings for men in recovery to share their experiences and receive support from others who understand the challenges of addiction.
- **Online Communities**: For those who may not have access to local support groups or prefer online resources, there are a variety of online communities and forums where men can connect with others in recovery.
- **Sober Living Houses**: These are residential homes where individuals in recovery can live in a drug-free environment while they work on their sobriety. Sober living houses offer a supportive, structured environment for individuals to transition from treatment to independent living.

3.3 Government and Non-Profit Organizations

- **Government Programs**: Many governments provide financial assistance and healthcare programs for individuals seeking treatment for substance abuse. This includes insurance coverage for rehabilitation programs and medication-assisted therapies.
- **Non-Profit Organizations**: Numerous non-profit organizations offer services such as counseling, recovery coaching, and educational programs to help men overcome substance abuse. They may also advocate for public policy changes to address substance abuse.

Chapter 12: Aging Gracefully: Health in Later Years

Introduction

Aging is an inevitable process that affects everyone, yet it is often misunderstood and associated with physical decline, diminished vitality, and loss of independence. However, modern science, healthcare, and lifestyle management have significantly altered how we approach aging. Aging Gracefully does not just refer to managing the aesthetic or external appearance but, more importantly, to ensuring mental, physical, and emotional well-being in the later years of life. This chapter addresses men's shared health concerns as they age, highlights the importance of maintaining an active lifestyle, and discusses effective strategies for healthy aging to help individuals live fuller, healthier lives well into their later years.

Section 1: Common Health Concerns as Men Age

As men age, they face unique health challenges that differ from those experienced by women, and these can significantly impact their quality of life. Aging is associated with the gradual decline of physical and mental faculties and an increased risk of certain chronic diseases. Understanding these health concerns allows for proactive measures and early interventions.

1.1 Cardiovascular Health

Cardiovascular diseases (CVD) are one of the leading causes of death among older men. With aging, the heart and blood vessels undergo structural and functional changes. Arteries may become stiffer, and blood pressure may increase, leading to hypertension, which is a significant risk factor for heart attacks, strokes, and heart failure. Men are generally at a higher risk for heart disease than women, particularly after middle age. Common cardiovascular issues include:

- **Hypertension (High Blood Pressure)**: Over time, the walls of the arteries lose elasticity, leading to higher blood pressure.
- **Atherosclerosis**: The buildup of plaque in the arteries can restrict blood flow, increasing the risk of heart attacks.
- **Heart Failure**: The heart's ability to pump blood efficiently decreases as muscle mass diminishes.

1.2 Musculoskeletal Health

Men experience a natural decline in muscle mass and bone density as they age. This can lead to a variety of musculoskeletal conditions, including:

- **Osteoarthritis**: The breakdown of cartilage in the joints leads to pain, swelling, and stiffness, especially in weight-bearing joints such as the knees, hips, and lower back.

- **Osteoporosis**: A condition where bones become brittle and fragile due to loss of bone mass, increasing the risk of fractures.
- **Muscle Loss (Sarcopenia)**: The natural decline in muscle mass and strength can make men more susceptible to falls and fractures.

Maintaining strength through regular exercise can help slow the progression of these conditions.

1.3 Mental Health

Mental health concerns become more prevalent with age, as men may face loneliness, cognitive decline, and emotional stress due to various life transitions. Common issues include:

- **Dementia and Alzheimer's Disease**: Cognitive decline is one of the most significant fears among aging men. These conditions can impair memory, reasoning, and daily functioning.
- **Depression**: Often underdiagnosed in older men, depression can manifest in various ways, such as irritability, lack of energy, and withdrawal from social activities.
- **Anxiety and Stress**: With aging, many men face stressors like retirement, the loss of loved ones, and health concerns, which can contribute to heightened anxiety levels.

Addressing mental health concerns is crucial for maintaining overall health and well-being.

1.4 Diabetes and Metabolic Health

Metabolic diseases, particularly diabetes, become more prevalent as men age. Age-related changes in metabolism and lifestyle factors like diet and physical activity contribute to the development of type 2 diabetes. Issues include:

- **Insulin Resistance**: As men age, their bodies may become less responsive to insulin, leading to higher blood sugar levels.
- **Obesity**: Increased body fat, particularly around the abdomen, is a significant risk factor for type 2 diabetes and other metabolic disorders.
- **Chronic Inflammation**: Aging is often accompanied by low-grade inflammation, which can worsen conditions like diabetes.

Managing blood sugar levels through diet, exercise, and, when necessary, medication can prevent the onset of diabetes or manage it effectively.

1.5 Prostate Health

The prostate gland often experiences changes with age, which can lead to several conditions:

- **Benign Prostatic Hyperplasia (BPH)**: As men age, the prostate may enlarge, leading to urinary symptoms such as frequent urination, urgency, and difficulty emptying the bladder.
- **Prostate Cancer**: Prostate cancer is the most common cancer among older men. While not all cases are life-threatening, early detection and treatment are essential.

Regular check-ups and screenings for prostate health are essential as part of a man's healthcare routine.

1.6 Sexual Health

Sexual health can be affected by various factors as men age, including hormonal changes, health conditions, and medications. Common concerns include:

- **Erectile Dysfunction (ED)**: As testosterone levels decline with age, erectile dysfunction becomes more common.
- **Low Testosterone**: Testosterone levels naturally decrease, leading to fatigue, reduced libido, and muscle loss.
- **Sexual Performance and Satisfaction**: Age-related physical and psychological changes can impact sexual satisfaction, which often requires communication and lifestyle adjustments.

Addressing sexual health concerns openly with healthcare providers can lead to effective treatments and solutions.

Section 2: The Importance of Maintaining an Active Lifestyle

An active lifestyle is one of the most critical factors in promoting health and longevity as men age. Regular physical activity helps mitigate many health risks associated with aging and is vital in maintaining mental and physical well-being.

2.1 Physical Activity and Cardiovascular Health

Regular exercise, particularly aerobic activities like walking, cycling, and swimming, helps improve heart health by:

- Reducing blood pressure.
- Improving circulation.
- Strengthening the heart and lungs.

Exercise has been shown to lower the risk of cardiovascular diseases, including heart attacks, strokes, and high cholesterol, by promoting the healthy functioning of the cardiovascular system.

2.2 Maintaining Muscle and Bone Health

Strength training and weight-bearing exercises prevent sarcopenia (muscle loss) and osteoporosis (bone thinning). Strengthening exercises help:

- Build muscle mass, which naturally declines with age.
- Maintain bone density, reducing the risk of fractures.
- Improve balance and coordination, decreasing the likelihood of falls.

Lifting weights, bodyweight exercises, or resistance training can benefit older men significantly.

2.3 Mental Health and Cognitive Function

Physical activity is also closely tied to mental well-being. Exercise helps manage stress and reduces the symptoms of depression and anxiety. Moreover, it has been shown to:

- Improve cognitive function, including memory and concentration.
- Reduce the risk of cognitive decline and dementia.
- Promote better sleep quality.

Regular physical activity is one of the most effective ways to prevent mental health issues and preserve brain health in later years.

2.4 Social Interaction and Emotional Well-Being

Exercise also provides opportunities for social interaction in group classes, sports, or community events. Social engagement has been shown to:

- Combat loneliness and isolation.
- Improve overall emotional health.
- Increase self-esteem and confidence.

Participating in active hobbies or community groups fosters a sense of belonging and purpose, both essential for aging.

Section 3: Strategies for Healthy Aging

Aging is about avoiding disease and maintaining an optimal quality of life. Several strategies focusing on physical, mental, and social well-being can help men age gracefully.

3.1 Nutrition and Diet

A well-balanced diet plays a crucial role in healthy aging. Proper nutrition can help prevent many age-related health problems, including obesity, diabetes, and cardiovascular disease. Key dietary guidelines for aging men include:

- **Balanced Macronutrients**: A diet rich in fruits, vegetables, whole grains, lean proteins, and healthy fats provides essential nutrients for energy, muscle maintenance, and immune function.
- **Calcium and Vitamin D**: These nutrients maintain strong bones and prevent osteoporosis.
- **Antioxidants**: Foods rich in antioxidants, such as berries, nuts, and leafy greens, help combat oxidative stress and promote cellular health.

- **Hydration**: Staying hydrated is essential for maintaining kidney health, digestion, and skin elasticity.

A proper diet, combined with the right supplements (under medical guidance), can enhance vitality and reduce the impact of aging on the body.

3.2 Regular Medical Check-ups and Screenings

Regular medical check-ups and screenings are among the best ways to ensure healthy aging. These helps detect potential issues early, when they are often easier to treat. Essential screenings for aging men include:

- **Blood Pressure Monitoring**: Early detection of hypertension allows for better management.
- **Cholesterol and Blood Sugar Tests**: Screening for high cholesterol and diabetes can prevent heart disease and metabolic disorders.
- **Prostate and Colon Cancer Screening**: Early detection of cancers through regular screenings (like PSA tests or colonoscopies) can improve treatment outcomes.
- **Vision and Hearing Tests**: Regular eye and ear exams help manage age-related sensory impairments.

3.3 Stress Management and Mental Health Care

As previously mentioned, mental health is a significant component of aging well. Effective stress management techniques include:

- **Mindfulness and Meditation**: These practices help reduce stress, improve focus, and enhance emotional well-being.
- **Social Engagement**: Connecting with family, friends, and community reduces feelings of isolation and fosters a sense of belonging.

Chapter 13: The Role of Mental Resilience

1.   **Understanding Mental Resilience and Its Benefits**

Mental resilience is adapting to and recovering from adversity, trauma, or significant stress. It involves coping with difficult situations, returning from challenges, and maintaining emotional stability and strength in the face of adversity. Resilient individuals do not just endure hardship but grow through it, learning valuable lessons that shape their future responses to stress.

Key Aspects of Mental Resilience:

- **Emotional Strength**: Resilience is often associated with emotional regulation. Resilient people can experience negative emotions, but don't let them control their lives. They can manage feelings like fear, frustration, and sadness without letting them undermine their well-being.
- **Adaptability**: Mental resilience involves flexibility in the face of adversity. People with high resilience are flexible in their approaches to problems. They can reassess their goals, plans, and strategies in response to changes or setbacks.
- **Optimism**: A resilient mindset is often linked to a sense of optimism. Resilient individuals maintain a hopeful outlook, believing that setbacks are temporary and that challenges can be overcome with effort and perseverance.
- **Self-Efficacy**: Resilience is closely tied to the belief in one's ability to influence events and outcomes in life. Resilient people often exhibit a strong sense of self-efficacy, which means they feel capable of managing their emotions, thoughts, and actions to navigate difficult situations.

Benefits of Mental Resilience:

- **Stress Reduction**: Resilience helps reduce the negative impact of stress on mental and physical health. Resilient individuals tend to experience less anxiety, depression, and other mental health issues because they can process stress more effectively.
- **Improved Coping Mechanisms**: Mentally resilient individuals use various coping strategies in challenging situations. These strategies help them deal with stress in ways that preserve their mental health and encourage positive outcomes.
- **Better Decision-Making**: People can think more clearly under pressure and are more resilient. They can approach challenges with a clearer mind, often leading to more sound decision-making.
- **Greater Sense of Control**: Building resilience leads to greater internal control and autonomy. Resilient individuals feel more empowered in managing their responses to challenging situations rather than being at the mercy of external circumstances.

- **Personal Growth**: Resilience helps people not just survive adversity but thrive. Overcoming challenges can lead to self-awareness, emotional intelligence, and personal strength growth.

1. **Techniques to Build Resilience: Coping Strategies and Positive Thinking**

While some aspects of mental resilience are innate, it is a skill that can be developed through practice. Several proven techniques for building resilience involve both cognitive and emotional strategies.

Coping Strategies:

- **Problem-Solving**: One of the most effective ways to build resilience is by learning to break problems down into manageable parts. This helps reduce the overwhelming feelings that come with significant challenges. Developing a systematic approach to problem-solving allows individuals to feel more in control and less stressed.
- **Mindfulness and Meditation**: Practicing mindfulness allows individuals to stay present and focused, which can help them avoid feeling overwhelmed by future or past events. Meditation helps clear the mind, reduce stress, and promote relaxation, all contributing to mental resilience.
- **Stress Management**: Learning how to identify and manage stress sources effectively is essential for building resilience. Techniques such as deep breathing, progressive muscle relaxation, and guided imagery can help reduce the body's physiological response to stress.
- **Time Management**: Effective time management reduces the feeling of being overwhelmed. By organizing daily tasks and setting realistic goals, individuals can build resilience by managing their workload without burning out.
- **Seeking Support**: Building resilience does not mean doing everything alone. Resilient people recognize when they need help and contact their support network. Emotional support from family, friends, or colleagues can help people process difficult emotions and share the burden of adversity.
- **Self-Care**: Physical health can bolster resilience. Regular exercise, healthy eating, adequate sleep, and engaging in activities that promote well-being (e.g., hobbies, relaxation techniques) all support mental resilience by maintaining overall health.
- **Gratitude Practice**: Focusing on positive aspects of life can improve mental resilience. By practicing gratitude, people can shift their focus away from problems and stressors toward positive life elements, fostering a more resilient mindset.
- **Developing a Growth Mindset**: Resilient people view challenges as opportunities for growth. Developing a growth mindset, where one

sees mistakes as learning experiences, helps people build resilience by transforming setbacks into stepping stones.

Positive Thinking:

- **Reframing**: Reframing involves changing the way an individual interprets a situation. Instead of viewing a problem as an insurmountable obstacle, reframing encourages seeing it as a challenge or opportunity for personal growth. This shift in perspective can help reduce anxiety and increase resilience.
- **Self-Talk**: Positive self-talk is a powerful tool for building mental resilience. It involves replacing negative, self-defeating thoughts with affirming, constructive thoughts. For example, replacing "I can't do this" with "I'll give this my best effort" can help boost confidence and reduce feelings of helplessness.
- **Affirmations**: Repeating positive affirmations helps reprogram the mind to focus on strengths and abilities rather than limitations. Simple affirmations like "I am strong" or "I can handle this" can cultivate a more resilient mindset.
- **Visualization**: Visualization involves imagining oneself succeeding under challenging situations. This mental practice helps individuals build confidence, feel more in control, and prepare mentally for challenges.
- **Acceptance**: Accepting that some things are beyond our control can reduce frustration and help build resilience. By focusing on what can be controlled (our actions, responses, and emotions), individuals can cope better with these situations.

1. **Personal Stories of Overcoming Challenges**

One of the most powerful ways to understand mental resilience is through real-life stories of individuals who have overcome significant adversity. These stories illustrate the transformative power of resilience and provide valuable lessons for others facing similar challenges.

Example 1: Overcoming Illness

Consider the story of a woman diagnosed with cancer at a young age. Initially, the diagnosis left her feeling helpless and devastated. However, she chose to focus on what she could control—her attitude, her treatment options, and her support network. She practiced mindfulness, sought emotional support from her family and friends, and kept a positive outlook despite the difficult circumstances. Throughout her treatment, she continued to work toward her professional goals and even became an advocate for cancer awareness. Her resilience not only helped her survive cancer but also turned her experience into an opportunity to help others facing similar battles.

Example 2: Rising After Job Loss

Another powerful example is an individual who faced a sudden job loss amid a personal crisis. Instead of succumbing to feelings of despair, they used the opportunity to reassess their skills, strengths, and passions. They turned to online learning and developed new skills, eventually leading to a new career path. This person's story highlights how resilience can help individuals bounce back from seemingly impossible setbacks and use challenges as stepping stones to tremendous success.

Example 3: A Personal Struggle with Mental Health

An individual facing a prolonged battle with mental health issues, such as depression or anxiety, might have initially felt overwhelmed by the thought of ever recovering. However, through therapy, self-care, and building a strong support system, they gradually learned to manage their emotions and thoughts more effectively. With time, they began to see setbacks as part of the recovery journey, and their resilience allowed them to maintain hope and work toward stability and well-being.

Example 4: The Journey of a Refugee

Consider the story of a refugee fleeing from a war-torn country. The challenges of displacement, loss of loved ones, and adapting to a new culture could have easily led to despair. However, this individual focused on rebuilding their life, learning a new language, and finding work. By leaning into their resilience, they created a new life for themselves and their family, proving that even in the darkest circumstances, the strength of the human spirit can prevail.

Conclusion

- Mental resilience is a crucial aspect of personal development and well-being. By understanding its benefits, practicing coping strategies, fostering positive thinking, and drawing inspiration from personal stories, individuals can build their resilience and navigate life's challenges with greater strength and adaptability. Resilience doesn't mean avoiding difficulties; instead, it's about embracing adversity and using it as a tool for growth. Whether managing stress, overcoming personal setbacks, or handling professional challenges, mental resilience is key to leading a fulfilling and successful life.

Chapter 14: The Impact of Technology on Health

Introduction: Technology has significantly transformed healthcare management and overall well-being. The advent of digital tools, devices, apps, and innovations in medical research has improved the ability to monitor health, prevent diseases, and support individuals in managing conditions. While these advancements offer many benefits, risks, and challenges are associated with their increasing reliance. This chapter delves into how technology impacts health, focusing on the pros and cons of health management, fitness, and nutrition apps, as well as the effects of screen time.

1. **The Pros and Cons of Technology in Health Management**

Pros:

1. **Improved Access to Healthcare:** Technology has democratized access to healthcare services. Telemedicine, for example, has allowed individuals to consult healthcare professionals from the comfort of their homes, especially in remote or underserved regions. Patients can now access specialist services that may have been previously unavailable due to geographic or financial constraints.

2. **Enhanced Monitoring and Tracking:** Wearable devices and remote health monitoring systems enable continuous tracking of health metrics, such as heart rate, blood pressure, sleep patterns, and physical activity levels. This data gives patients and healthcare providers real-time insights into health conditions, enabling quicker responses to health issues. The ability to track chronic conditions like diabetes or hypertension is a significant breakthrough in managing long-term health.

3. **Personalized Treatment and Preventive Care:** Thanks to technology, healthcare providers can now tailor treatment plans to patients' unique needs. Data from genetic testing, lifestyle habits, and ongoing health monitoring enable more personalized care. Preventive care has also become more effective, as health apps and digital tools provide reminders for medical check-ups, vaccinations, and healthy lifestyle changes.

4. **Increased Efficiency in Health Systems:** Electronic Health Records (EHRs) have revolutionized how medical data is stored, accessed, and shared. This has streamlined administrative processes, improved the accuracy of patient records, and reduced the risk of medical errors. Moreover, technology has facilitated quicker diagnoses through advanced imaging technologies and AI-assisted diagnostics.

5. **Better Health Education and Awareness:** Digital platforms offer accessible health education, empowering individuals to make informed decisions about their well-being. People can access a wealth

of information about diseases, preventive measures, fitness routines, and mental health strategies from websites to social media. Public health campaigns often leverage these technologies to raise awareness about important health issues like vaccination and mental health.

Cons:

1. **Over-Reliance on Technology:** While technology can aid in health management, there is a risk of over-reliance. Patients may rely more on devices and apps for diagnoses and treatment recommendations rather than consulting healthcare professionals. Misinterpreting data from health apps or wearables can lead to false reassurance or unwarranted panic.

2. **Privacy and Security Risks:** Digitalizing health data raises concerns about privacy and security. Personal health information is highly sensitive, and breaches of this data can have serious consequences. While healthcare providers and tech companies take measures to safeguard this information, the risk of hacking and unauthorized access remains a significant challenge.

3. **Digital Divide:** Only some have equal access to the latest technologies, especially in low-income or rural areas. The digital divide exacerbates healthcare inequalities, as those with access to smartphones, high-speed internet, or modern devices may be included in digital health advancements. Additionally, older adults or those with limited digital literacy may need help to use health technology effectively.

4. **Potential Negative Impact on Physical and Mental Health:** The extensive use of technology, particularly smartphones and computers, can contribute to physical health issues such as eye strain, poor posture, and lack of physical activity. Additionally, excessive screen time is linked to mental health challenges, including anxiety, depression, and poor sleep quality. The constant connectivity may lead to burnout and stress, undermining the very health improvements technology is meant to support.

5. **Cost Implications:** High-tech health devices and software solutions often incur substantial costs. While some health apps are free, many of the most effective and comprehensive tools require premium subscriptions or initial investments in hardware (such as wearables). This can create barriers for individuals who need help to afford these technologies, potentially limiting their access to the benefits of digital health.

6. **Apps and Tools for Fitness and Nutrition Tracking**

Overview: Fitness and nutrition tracking apps have surged in popularity, providing individuals with the tools to monitor their physical activity and nutritional intake. These apps help users set goals, track progress, and make data-driven decisions about their health. The benefits and challenges of these apps are critical to understand in the context of overall health management.

1. **Fitness Tracking Apps:** Fitness tracking apps monitor physical activity, from simple step-counting to more detailed tracking of exercise routines, calories burned, and heart rate. Popular apps like Fitbit, Strava, and MyFitnessPal track daily steps and workouts and provide insights into users' overall fitness levels. These apps typically sync with wearable devices that track data, including smartwatches and fitness bands, offering real-time feedback.

2. **Benefits:**
   - **Goal Setting and Motivation:** Fitness apps help users set specific goals such as daily steps, calories burned, or workouts completed. The sense of achievement after meeting these goals can motivate individuals to remain active.
   - **Personalized Recommendations:** Many apps provide customized workout plans based on user preferences and fitness levels. With AI technology, these apps evolve with the user's progress, recommending changes to exercise routines or introducing new challenges to keep the experience fresh and motivating.
   - **Community and Social Sharing:** Fitness apps often have social features, allowing users to share their achievements and progress with friends or community groups. This fosters a sense of accountability and can encourage friendly competition, further motivating individuals to stay on track.

3. **Challenges:**
   - **Accuracy Issues:** While fitness trackers provide valuable data, their accuracy can vary. Step counts or calorie burn estimates may sometimes be vague, and over-reliance on these metrics could mislead users.
   - **Addiction to Tracking:** The constant monitoring of fitness data can lead to an obsession with numbers, potentially causing anxiety or negative body image issues. Some individuals may become overly focused on tracking, neglecting holistic well-being.

4. **Nutrition Tracking Apps:** Nutrition apps, such as MyFitnessPal, Lose It! and Chronometer, enable users to log their meals and monitor their nutritional intake. These apps typically feature databases of food items and their nutritional values, helping individuals understand how their diet aligns with their health goals.

5. **Benefits:**

- **Awareness and Education:** Nutrition apps help users become more mindful of what they are eating by showing the nutritional content of food. This can lead to healthier eating habits and better decision-making regarding meal planning.

- **Customizable Goals:** Many nutrition apps allow users to set specific dietary goals, such as reducing sugar intake or increasing protein consumption, making it easier to stay on track with personalized health objectives.

- **Integration with Fitness Apps:** Many nutrition and fitness apps can sync data, providing a comprehensive view of a person's health. For example, users can track calories consumed and burned, helping to achieve weight loss or muscle gain goals.

6. **Challenges:**

- **Inaccuracy in Food Logging:** While food databases are extensive, there may be discrepancies in the nutritional values of specific foods or portion sizes. Users may also inaccurately estimate portions, leading to underreporting or overreporting of calorie intake.

- **Overemphasis on Numbers:** Just like fitness tracking, some individuals may become fixated on numbers, potentially leading to unhealthy eating behaviors or restrictive dieting.

7. **Managing Screen Time and Its Effects on Health**

Overview: As digital technology continues to be integrated into every aspect of daily life, managing screen time has become a critical health concern. Prolonged screen exposure can negatively affect physical and mental well-being, but technology also offers solutions to help individuals monitor and reduce screen time.

1. **Physical Effects of Excessive Screen Time:**

- **Eye Strain and Dry Eyes:** Prolonged screen use can cause discomfort, known as "digital eye strain," characterized by dry eyes, headaches, and blurry vision.

- **Posture Issues:** Excessive screen time, especially when using devices in improper postures, can lead to neck, back, and shoulder pain. This is often referred to as "tech neck."

- **Sleep Disruption:** Screens emit blue light, especially before bedtime, which can disrupt circadian rhythms and affect sleep quality, leading to sleep deprivation and fatigue.

2. **Mental and Emotional Health Concerns:**

    - **Increased Stress and Anxiety:** Constant screen use, mainly social media, can contribute to feelings of anxiety, stress, and depression. Comparing oneself to others online, cyberbullying, and information overload are all factors that can negatively impact mental health.

    - **Reduced Social Interaction:** Prolonged screen use, particularly in isolation, may reduce face-to-face interactions, contributing to loneliness and disconnection from the real world.

3. **Technology Solutions for Managing Screen Time:**

    - **Screen Time Tracking Apps:** Many mobile devices have built-in screen time management tools. These apps allow users to track how much time they spend on various apps and set usage limits.

    - **Blue Light Filters:** Devices can be equipped with blue light filters, or users can install software that reduces blue light emission during nighttime hours to help

Chapter 15: Nutrition Myths Debunked

Nutrition is essential to overall health, yet many misconceptions about what constitutes a healthy diet persist. This chapter aims to clarify some of the most common myths about men's nutrition, provide evidence-based insights into making informed dietary choices, and offer guidance on navigating the conflicting health advice that often circulates in popular media and on social platforms.

1. **Common Misconceptions About Men's Nutrition**

Men's nutrition is often surrounded by myths and misconceptions. These myths are perpetuated by outdated dietary guidelines, food company marketing, and misinformation in the media. In this section, we'll debunk some of the most common nutrition myths targeting men and their health.

1.1 Myth #1: Men Need a High-Protein Diet to Build Muscle

Many assume that high protein intake is the most critical muscle-building factor. While protein is essential for muscle repair and growth, excessive amounts are unnecessary and can be harmful in the long run. Studies show that men (and women) need about 1.6 to 2.2 grams of protein per kilogram of body weight per day to support muscle building, and going above this level only sometimes results in more significant muscle growth. A balanced diet with sufficient carbohydrates and fats is crucial for maintaining overall health and muscle performance.

1.2 Myth #2: Men Should Avoid Carbs for Weight Loss

Various weight loss programs have popularized low-carb diets, but the idea that men should altogether avoid carbs to lose weight is misleading. Carbohydrates are a primary energy source, and when consumed in appropriate amounts, they play an essential role in metabolic processes, including hormone regulation, brain function, and exercise performance. The key is choosing healthy, unprocessed carbs, such as whole grains, vegetables, and fruits, rather than refined sugars and processed foods.

1.3 Myth #3: Fat is Bad for You and Leads to Heart Disease

The myth that all fats are bad and should be avoided persists in many popular diets. However, research has shown that not all fats are created equal. Unsaturated fats in foods like olive oil, nuts, avocados, and fatty fish benefit heart health. These fats help regulate cholesterol levels and provide essential fatty acids that the body cannot produce alone. On the other hand, trans fats and excessive saturated fats, often found in processed foods, can contribute to heart disease and should be limited.

1.4 Myth #4: Supplements Are Necessary for Optimal Health

Many men believe that taking various supplements—such as multivitamins, protein powders, and testosterone boosters—is essential for good health. A balanced diet rich in whole foods should provide most of the nutrients the body needs. Supplements may be helpful for those with specific deficiencies in some cases, but they should never replace real food. Overreliance on supplements can also lead to imbalances and even toxicity.

1.5 Myth #5: Men Can't Be Vegetarians or Vegans and Still Build Muscle

It's a common misconception that men need meat to build Muscle and that plant-based diets are insufficient. However, numerous professional athletes and bodybuilders follow plant-based diets and thrive. A well-planned vegetarian or vegan diet can provide all the necessary protein, iron, calcium, and other nutrients to build Muscle. The key is to incorporate a variety of plant-based protein sources, such as beans, lentils, tofu, tempeh, quinoa, and nuts, and to ensure adequate intake of vitamins and minerals through food and possibly supplementation if needed.

1. **Evidence-Based Information to Guide Dietary Choices**

In this section, we will provide solid, evidence-based nutritional advice that men can follow to make informed and healthy dietary choices.

2.1 The Importance of a Balanced Diet

A balanced diet is fundamental to maintaining optimal health. Research consistently shows that various whole foods from different food groups, such as vegetables, fruits, whole grains, lean proteins, and healthy fats, are essential for preventing chronic diseases and promoting well-being. Men's daily caloric intake should be adjusted based on their age, activity level, and health goals, but on average, adult men require 2,000 to 3,000 calories per day. A balanced diet provides necessary nutrients and helps manage weight, improve mental clarity, and boost energy levels.

2.2 Macronutrients: Carbs, Proteins, and Fats

Understanding the role of macronutrients—carbohydrates, proteins, and fats—is critical to making informed dietary choices.

- **Carbohydrates** are the body's preferred energy source, especially for brain function and exercise. Choosing complex carbohydrates, such as whole grains, vegetables, and fruits, ensures the body receives fiber and essential nutrients.
- **Proteins** are crucial for muscle repair, immune function, and enzyme production. In addition to meat, other high-quality protein sources include dairy products, legumes, and plant-based proteins like tofu and tempeh.
- **Fats** are necessary for hormone production, cellular structure, and energy. Focus on healthy fats from sources like fish, nuts, seeds, and plant oils while avoiding excessive saturated and trans fats.

2.3 Micronutrients: Vitamins and Minerals

Micronutrients are vital to overall health, and while they are required in smaller amounts than macronutrients, they are no less important. Vitamins such as vitamin D, B12, and C and minerals like magnesium, calcium, and zinc support immune function, muscle contraction, bone health, and cognitive function. Many micronutrient deficiencies can be addressed with a balanced, nutrient-rich diet. For example, leafy greens, nuts, seeds, and legumes are excellent sources of magnesium, while fruits and vegetables provide high amounts of vitamins and antioxidants.

2.4 Hydration: The Key to Good Health

Staying hydrated is often overlooked, but it's a crucial aspect of nutrition. Proper hydration supports digestive function, kidney health, and cognitive function. Men should aim to drink at least 3.7 liters (125 ounces) of water daily, depending on activity level and climate. Coffee, tea, and water-rich foods like fruits and vegetables can contribute to hydration, but sugary drinks should be avoided.

2.5 Nutritional Timing: Eating for Performance and Recovery

Proper nutrition timing can enhance performance, recovery, and overall health for active men. Eating enough throughout the day supports energy needs, especially before and after exercise. Consuming protein and carbohydrates, post-workout can help repair muscles and replenish glycogen stores, accelerating recovery. Research also suggests that spreading protein intake across meals can optimize muscle protein synthesis rather than consuming large amounts in one sitting.

1.   **How to Navigate Conflicting Health Advice**

In the age of social media and constant health trends, conflicting nutrition advice can be overwhelming. Navigating this sea of information requires critical thinking and understanding how to evaluate health claims.

3.1 Identifying Reliable Sources of Information

The first step in navigating conflicting advice is to identify trustworthy sources of information. Peer-reviewed scientific journals, accredited health organizations like the World Health Organization (WHO) or the National Institutes of Health (NIH), and certified nutritionists or dietitians are credible sources. On the other hand, anecdotal advice from unqualified individuals or sources with commercial interests (e.g., supplement companies) should be viewed with skepticism.

3.2 Recognizing Red Flags in Health Advice

Not all health advice is created equal, and some red flags can indicate misinformation. Be wary of:

- **Promises of quick fixes** (e.g., "lose 10 pounds in 10 days").
- **Claims of miracle foods or supplements** that promise to cure diseases or boost performance without evidence.
- **Excessive reliance on testimonials** instead of scientific data.
- **Extreme diets** that eliminate entire food groups without a clear, evidence-based rationale.

3.3 Understanding the Role of Individual Differences

Nutrition is not one-size-fits-all. Factors such as age, gender, genetics, activity level, and preexisting health conditions all affect how the body responds to different foods. What works for one person may not work for another, so personalized nutrition, possibly with the help of a registered dietitian, is increasingly being recognized as a more practical approach.

3.4 Keeping an Open Mind While Sticking to the Evidence

While being open to new information is essential, sticking to proven, evidence-based practices is equally crucial. The latest trends and research will continue to emerge, but foundational principles such as eating a balanced diet rich in whole foods remain the cornerstone of good nutrition. It's essential to evaluate new information critically and resist jumping to conclusions based on the latest fad.

3.5 The Importance of Long-Term Health over Short-Term Trends

Finally, men should prioritize long-term health goals over short-term trends. Focusing on sustainable, realistic dietary habits rather than following the latest fad diets ensures better health outcomes in the future. Nutritional choices should support overall wellness, including mental health, energy, immune function, and chronic disease prevention, rather than providing quick fixes for temporary goals.

Conclusion

Nutrition is complex, but separating fact from myth can help men make informed dietary choices that lead to better health outcomes. By debunking common misconceptions, understanding the science behind nutrition, and learning how to navigate conflicting advice, men can optimize their diets for

Chapter 16: The Power of Community and Support Groups

Introduction to Community Support in Health and Well-being

The human experience is deeply rooted in connection, shared experiences, and support systems. Whether facing a chronic illness, going through a significant life change, or striving for a healthier lifestyle, the role of communities and support groups cannot be overstated. Communities focused on health and well-being offer individuals a sense of belonging, shared wisdom, and a collective strength that often surpasses individual efforts. This chapter explores the benefits of joining health-focused communities, how to find local and online support groups, and personal stories of transformation that highlight the power of these supportive networks.

Benefits of Joining Health-Focused Communities

1. Emotional and Psychological Support

One of the most significant benefits of joining health-focused communities is the emotional support they provide. Health challenges, whether physical or mental, can lead to feelings of isolation, fear, and helplessness. Being part of a community allows individuals to share their struggles and receive empathy from others who understand their situation. This mutual support helps reduce feelings of loneliness, anxiety, and depression, which can often accompany health issues.

Support groups foster an environment where individuals can openly express their emotions without fear of judgment. This emotional release is crucial for mental well-being and can significantly improve one's overall outlook on life. Studies have shown that social support can reduce the impact of stress, enhance coping mechanisms, and even improve immune function.

1. Information Sharing and Knowledge Exchange

Whether online or offline, health-focused communities often provide a wealth of information about managing illnesses, adopting healthier lifestyles, or navigating healthcare systems. Members of these communities share personal experiences, advice, and resources, which can be invaluable in making informed decisions. For example, individuals dealing with chronic conditions like diabetes, arthritis, or cancer can exchange tips on medication management, dietary recommendations, or coping strategies.

Moreover, health professionals or experts occasionally participate in these communities, providing trusted, evidence-based guidance. This exchange of information helps individuals stay informed about the latest treatments, therapies, and health practices.

1. **Motivation and Accountability**

Another significant benefit is the motivation and accountability of being part of a group. Members of a health-focused community often have similar goals, such as weight loss, quitting smoking, or managing a specific health condition. Having a network of people working toward similar objectives can inspire individuals to stay committed to their health goals. Regular check-ins, progress tracking, and positive reinforcement from group members can help individuals stay motivated and hold themselves accountable.

In fact, research has shown that people who participate in support groups tend to succeed more in maintaining lifestyle changes, such as improved nutrition, regular exercise, or adherence to treatment plans, than those who try to manage their health challenges in isolation.

1. **Sense of Belonging and Reduced Stigma**

Health challenges, particularly mental health conditions, can often be stigmatized in society. Many individuals feel ashamed or embarrassed about their health issues, which may prevent them from seeking help or talking about their struggles. However, being part of a community can normalize these experiences and help reduce stigma.

In a health-focused group, individuals are reminded that they are not alone in their struggles. This sense of belonging and understanding can foster acceptance and self-compassion. The community becomes a safe space where individuals can share their vulnerabilities without fear of judgment or discrimination.

Finding Local and Online Support Groups

1. **Locating Local Support Groups**

Finding local support groups is essential in connecting with a community that can offer the emotional and practical support needed. Many hospitals, healthcare centers, and non-profit organizations host or facilitate support groups for patients with specific health issues. These groups often meet regularly and are led by trained facilitators, counselors, or healthcare professionals.

- **Hospitals and Healthcare Facilities:** Many hospitals offer support groups for patients with chronic illnesses, mental health disorders, or those recovering from surgeries. These groups are often led by social workers, psychologists, or patient care coordinators who provide a structured environment for discussion and peer support.
- **Non-Profit Organizations:** Various organizations focused on specific health conditions (e.g., cancer, diabetes, mental health) often host support groups. These groups are valuable for meeting others who are going through similar experiences.
- **Community Centers and Libraries:** Local community centers or libraries may offer support groups for different health issues. These are often free or low-cost and provide opportunities to meet in person.

Finding a local support group often involves contacting healthcare providers, non-profit organizations, or community centers. Additionally, speaking with a social worker or healthcare team may provide recommendations for nearby groups.

1. **Online Support Groups**

In today's digital age, online support groups offer a convenient and often more accessible alternative to in-person meetings. These groups connect individuals worldwide, allowing them to share their experiences and support one another without geographical constraints. Online communities can be particularly beneficial for individuals in rural or remote areas, those with mobility issues, or anyone seeking anonymity.

- **Social Media and Forums:** Platforms like Facebook, Reddit, and specialized forums host numerous health-related groups individuals can join based on their specific conditions or interests. These groups are typically private or closed, ensuring members can discuss sensitive topics safely.
- **Health Websites and Apps:** Websites dedicated to specific health conditions often host forums or online support groups. Additionally, many health apps have built-in community features that allow users to connect with others facing similar challenges.
- **Telemedicine Platforms:** Many healthcare providers and organizations now offer virtual support groups or therapy sessions

through telemedicine platforms, making it easier for individuals to access support from home.

The flexibility of online support groups—especially for those with busy schedules or who live far from in-person options—has made them an increasingly popular choice for many people seeking support.

Personal Stories of Transformation Through Community Support

1. **Story of Recovery: Jenny's Battle with Cancer**

Jenny, a 42-year-old woman, was diagnosed with breast cancer. Her world turned upside down as she navigated the emotional and physical toll of her diagnosis and treatments. Initially, Jenny felt isolated and overwhelmed by the uncertainty of her future. However, after being introduced to a local cancer support group, she found a renewed sense of hope.

In this group, Jenny met other women going through similar experiences. They shared stories of their struggles, successes, and coping mechanisms. The group's support helped her feel understood and less alone. As she went through her chemotherapy treatments, she was motivated by the stories of other women who had come out the other side of their battles. The emotional support provided by the group was invaluable, and Jenny found herself more resilient and determined.

Jenny also learned practical advice through the support group on managing side effects, maintaining a positive mindset, and connecting with healthcare professionals. She credits the group as a cornerstone in her recovery, helping her face each day with strength and purpose.

1. **Transformation Through Online Support: Mark's Journey with Anxiety**

Mark had long struggled with anxiety and depression. He tried various treatments, but nothing seemed to provide lasting relief. He felt disconnected from his friends and family, unable to communicate the depth of his emotional pain. After a brutal episode, Mark searched for online mental health communities. He found a Facebook group specifically for individuals struggling with anxiety, and he decided to join.

At first, Mark was hesitant to share his experiences. However, he quickly realized that he was not alone. The group members were open, kind, and nonjudgmental. They shared similar experiences, and Mark found comfort in knowing that others understood the weight of living with anxiety.

Over time, Mark became an active group member, offering advice, support, and encouragement to others. Helping others gave him a sense of purpose and helped him manage his own mental health more effectively. The connections he made in the group gave him the courage to seek professional help, and he credits his involvement in the community for playing a significant role in his ongoing recovery.

1. **A Shared Journey: Maria's Weight Loss Success**

Maria, a 35-year-old mother of two, had struggled with her weight for many years. She had tried various diets and exercise programs, but nothing seemed to work. Feeling discouraged, she joined an online support group for women focused on weight loss and healthy living. In this group, Maria found a wealth of advice, encouragement, and personal stories of success.

The women in the group shared tips on meal planning, workouts, and staying motivated. More importantly, they shared their challenges and setbacks, making Maria feel less like a failure for struggling with her weight. She learned that weight loss wasn't just about dieting—it was about building a sustainable lifestyle, complete with support, self-compassion, and gradual progress.

Maria's journey took time, but with the support of her online community, she stayed focused and committed. Over a year, Maria lost over 40 pounds and developed a healthier, more balanced relationship with food and exercise. She credits the group's encouragement and shared experiences as essential to her success.

Conclusion: The Lifelong Benefits of Community Support

The power of community and support groups cannot be underestimated in terms of health and well-being. Whether online or in person, these communities provide a unique opportunity for individuals to find comfort, share knowledge, gain motivation, and connect with others who understand their struggles. The personal stories of transformation shared in this chapter highlight how impactful community support can be in overcoming health challenges.

Health-focused communities help individuals lead healthier, more fulfilling lives by fostering a sense of belonging, reducing stigma, and encouraging accountability.

Chapter 17: Integrating Mindfulness into Daily Life

Introduction

The chapter begins with an introduction to mindfulness, emphasizing its importance as a practice far beyond meditation. It explores how mindfulness can improve mental and physical health when integrated into daily life. The benefits of mindfulness will be explained in the context of its application to everyday activities and its long-term positive impact on the body and mind.

1. **The Benefits of Mindfulness for Mental and Physical Health**

1.1 Mental Health Benefits

Mindfulness can provide numerous mental health benefits, contributing to emotional well-being, stress reduction, and improved cognitive function. Key benefits include:

- **Stress Reduction**: Mindfulness helps manage and reduce stress by promoting relaxation and focusing attention. Mindfulness practices activate the parasympathetic nervous system (rest and digest), helping counteract the fight-or-flight response.
- **Enhanced Emotional Regulation**: Practicing mindfulness improves emotional awareness, allowing individuals to respond to emotional triggers rather than react impulsively. This regulation helps in managing anxiety, depression, and negative emotions more effectively.
- **Improved Focus and Attention**: Mindfulness encourages present-moment awareness, which enhances concentration and helps with focus. This is particularly beneficial in today's world of constant distractions.
- **Cognitive Flexibility**: Mindfulness can help cultivate cognitive flexibility, enabling individuals to shift their thinking patterns and perspectives. This ability can reduce rigid thinking and foster problem-solving skills.
- **Improved Self-awareness**: Mindfulness enhances self-awareness by paying attention to one's thoughts, feelings, and bodily sensations. This can lead to a deeper understanding of oneself and personal growth.

1.2 Physical Health Benefits

Mindfulness practices don't just benefit the mind; they can also significantly positively affect the body.

- **Reduced Blood Pressure**: Regular mindfulness practice has been shown to lower blood pressure and improve heart health by reducing stress and inducing a state of calmness.
- **Enhanced Immune Function**: Mindfulness has been linked to improved immune function, as it helps reduce stress hormones like cortisol, which, when elevated, can suppress the immune system.

- **Pain Management**: Mindfulness can change how the brain perceives and responds to pain. Studies show that mindfulness-based pain management techniques can reduce pain perception, help individuals cope better with chronic pain, and lower the need for medication.
- **Improved Sleep Quality**: Mindfulness helps regulate the body's stress response, allowing for better sleep. Reducing stress hormones leads to better sleep quality, assisting individuals in falling asleep faster and staying asleep longer.
- **Increased Physical Relaxation**: Through mindfulness practices like body scans or mindful breathing, individuals learn to release physical tension, reduce muscle stiffness, and improve overall body awareness.

1. **Simple Mindfulness Practices to Incorporate into Daily Routines**

The chapter will then dive into practical, simple mindfulness techniques that can easily be woven into daily life. These practices do not require any exceptional environment or extended time commitment, making them accessible for anyone to use.

2.1 Mindful Breathing

Mindful breathing is one of the simplest and most effective mindfulness practices. It involves paying attention to the breath entering and exiting the body. The focus should be on the sensations of the breath, such as the rise and fall of the chest or abdomen or the feeling of air entering the nostrils.

- **When to Practice**: Anytime throughout the day—while commuting, before a meeting, or during moments of stress.
- **How to Practice**: Take slow, deep breaths through the nose, hold for a moment, and then exhale slowly through the mouth. Notice the sensations of the breath and bring attention back to the breath if the mind wanders.

2.2 Mindful Eating

Mindful eating involves paying full attention to the act of eating. This practice encourages eating slowly, savoring each bite, and noticing food's textures, flavors and smells.

- **When to Practice**: During every meal, even snacks.
- **How to Practice**: Take a few deep breaths to calm the mind before eating. As you eat, try to chew slowly, paying attention to the taste and texture of the food. Avoid distractions like screens or multitasking while eating.

2.3 Mindful Walking

Mindful walking is a practice that combines physical movement with mindfulness. It involves strolling, focusing on each step, and noticing the sensations of the feet as they make contact with the ground.

- **When to Practice**: During a walk around the neighborhood, in nature, or inside your home or office.
- **How to Practice**: As you walk, become aware of your body's movements, the sensation of your feet touching the ground, and the environment around you. Stay present with each step, noticing how your body feels as it moves.

2.4 Body Scan

A body scan is a mindfulness technique that systematically scans the body to notice any sensations of tension or discomfort. The goal is to bring awareness to the body without judgment.

- **When to Practice**: Before bed or during moments of physical discomfort.
- **How to Practice**: Begin by lying or sitting comfortably. Close your eyes and focus on your breath. Start with your toes and slowly move up the body, paying attention to each part and noting any sensations. Gently release tension as you breathe in and out.

2.5 Mindful Listening

Mindful listening is about being fully present when listening to someone else, without distractions or judgments.

- **When to Practice**: During conversations or meetings.
- **How to Practice**: Listen attentively to the speaker, focusing on their words and tone without planning your response. Notice your reactions, but return your attention to the speaker, allowing them to feel heard.

2.6 Mindful Moments at Work

Workplaces can be stressful, but mindfulness can be incorporated into work routines to improve productivity and well-being.

- **When to Practice**: During breaks, before meetings, or when feeling overwhelmed.
- **How to Practice**: Take a few moments to pause and breathe deeply, focusing solely on your breath. Alternatively, briefly walk to reset and return to your tasks with a fresh perspective.

2.7 Mindful Technology Use

Technology can often lead to distractions and mental clutter. Mindful technology use involves using devices consciously and with purpose.

- **When to Practice**: Using phones, computers, or other digital devices.

- **How to Practice**: Set clear intentions for your use of technology. Avoid mindlessly scrolling or multitasking. Take short breaks to rest your eyes and mind.

1. **Personal Anecdotes of Mindfulness Success**

Personal anecdotes or success stories can be shared to make mindfulness feel more relatable and authentic. These stories demonstrate how mindfulness has transformed lives in real-world situations, making it more accessible to readers.

3.1 Story 1: Overcoming Anxiety at Work

A personal story about an individual who incorporated mindfulness techniques, such as mindful breathing and body scans, to manage workplace anxiety. This person shares how mindfulness helped them stay calm during high-pressure meetings and improved their productivity.

3.2 Story 2: Managing Chronic Pain with Mindfulness

A personal account from someone who suffered from chronic pain and used mindfulness to manage discomfort. The story illustrates how the individual used mindfulness practices, like mindful breathing and the body scan, to reduce their reliance on medication and improve their quality of life.

3.3 Story 3: Mindfulness for Better Sleep

A story of someone who struggled with insomnia and found relief through mindfulness practices. By practicing mindful breathing before bed and setting a calming routine, they improved their sleep quality and reduced nighttime anxiety.

3.4 Story 4: Mindfulness in Parenting

A parent shares their experience of using mindfulness techniques to stay present with their children, even during challenging moments. These techniques include mindful listening and breathing exercises to manage stress and improve interactions with their children.

3.5 Story 5: From Overwhelm to Calm: A Student's Journey

A student shares how mindfulness helped them manage academic stress, improve focus, and stay calm during exams. The student discusses their journey from feeling overwhelmed to experiencing a sense of balance and control.

Conclusion

The chapter concludes by reinforcing the importance of integrating mindfulness into daily life. It reminds readers that mindfulness is a practice and a way of living. By incorporating even a few simple mindfulness techniques into daily routines, individuals can experience mental and physical health improvements. The chapter ends with an encouraging message to begin small and gradually build a sustainable mindfulness practice that suits each individual's lifestyle.

Chapter 18: The Role of Hobbies and Interests

Introduction

In today's fast-paced world, where the demands of work, family, and societal expectations often dominate, it is easy to overlook the importance of hobbies and personal interests. Yet, these activities play a crucial role in contributing to mental, emotional, and physical well-being. This chapter delves into the multifaceted role of hobbies and interests in enhancing overall well-being, exploring the cognitive benefits of pursuing new interests, and discussing the art of balancing work, life, and leisure. By the end of this chapter, the reader will understand how engaging in hobbies and cultivating new interests can help achieve a balanced and fulfilling life.

Section 1: How Hobbies Contribute to Overall Well-Being

Hobbies are more than just ways to pass the time. They are vital to maintaining and enhancing well-being, ranging from emotional health to cognitive development. This section explores these benefits in detail.

1.1. Psychological Benefits of Hobbies

Stress relief is one of the most significant psychological benefits of engaging in hobbies. In today's world, where many individuals face constant pressure from work or personal responsibilities, hobbies provide a much-needed escape. Activities such as painting, gardening, knitting, or even playing video games can serve as a form of mindfulness, where individuals focus entirely on the present moment, free from worries about deadlines or other pressures. This immersion process helps lower cortisol levels, the hormone associated with stress, and can significantly improve mood.

Moreover, hobbies foster a sense of achievement and self-esteem. Whether mastering a musical instrument, completing a jigsaw puzzle, or growing a beautiful garden, hobbies offer individuals an opportunity to develop new skills, set goals, and witness progress. Setting and achieving personal goals outside of work provides a sense of accomplishment and enhances one's self-worth.

1.2. Emotional Health and Hobbies

Engaging in activities that bring joy can help mitigate feelings of anxiety, depression, and loneliness. For example, social hobbies like team sports, book clubs, or volunteer work help to cultivate a sense of belonging, combatting isolation. These social interactions foster supportive networks of friends and peers, contributing to emotional well-being. Even solitary hobbies like reading or crafting provide emotional fulfillment by offering a safe space for self-expression and creativity.

Moreover, research has shown that writing in journals or engaging in art therapy can be an outlet for emotions. This form of creative expression allows individuals to process their feelings productively, reducing the likelihood of emotional bottling and subsequent emotional outbursts.

1.3. Cognitive and Mental Health Benefits

Hobbies stimulate the brain, leading to cognitive benefits that improve mental health. Engaging in mentally challenging activities like playing chess, solving puzzles, or learning a new language keeps the mind sharp and enhances cognitive function. Studies have shown that older adults who engage in cognitively stimulating hobbies tend to experience slower mental decline compared to those who lead sedentary or unstimulated lifestyles. These activities promote neural plasticity, the brain's ability to form new neural connections, thereby maintaining mental agility.

Furthermore, hobbies can enhance memory retention. For instance, hobbies that involve remembering sequences, such as dancing or learning new recipes, can improve short-term and long-term memory.

1.4. Physical Health and Well-Being

Although hobbies are often considered mental or emotional, many also have physical benefits. Physical hobbies, such as yoga, hiking, cycling, or swimming, provide exercise that improves cardiovascular health, strengthen muscles, and boosts energy levels. Regular engagement in physical activities also reduces the risk of chronic diseases like heart disease, diabetes, and obesity.

Even sedentary hobbies like knitting, gardening, or drawing can improve physical well-being by enhancing fine motor skills and reducing tension. Due to their calming effect, engaging in hobbies can lower blood pressure, reduce the risk of heart disease, and improve sleep patterns.

Section 2: Exploring New Interests for Mental Stimulation

While established hobbies are beneficial, exploring new interests is equally important. Constantly learning and engaging in new activities stimulates the brain and helps break the monotony of daily routines. This section discusses how trying new hobbies can contribute to mental stimulation and personal growth.

2.1. The Importance of Lifelong Learning

Lifelong learning is the continuous, voluntary pursuit of knowledge for personal or professional development. Exploring new hobbies and interests is a key component of lifelong learning. Whether learning a new language, playing an instrument, or taking up photography, learning new things contributes to mental agility, creativity, and self-improvement.

New interests challenge the brain to adapt to unfamiliar concepts, skills, and ways of thinking. This type of mental stimulation is significant as individuals age. Research has shown that older adults who engage in new learning experiences have a lower risk of cognitive decline and dementia. Engaging in varied, challenging activities can help individuals stay mentally sharp for years.

2.2. Embracing Change and Adaptability

Trying new hobbies can foster adaptability, a crucial skill in an ever-changing world. Exploring different interests forces individuals to leave their comfort zones and embrace change. For example, learning a new sport or engaging in a new cultural activity encourages individuals to adopt new perspectives and thinking methods. This flexibility helps individuals become more resilient when faced with unexpected challenges or changes in their personal or professional lives.

Additionally, learning new things often requires problem-solving, which can enhance cognitive flexibility. People constantly acquiring new skills are better equipped to think critically, adapt to change, and handle life's uncertainties.

2.3. Social Benefits of Exploring New Interests

New interests can also offer opportunities for social connection. Joining a class, group, or online community to learn something new opens the door to meeting like-minded people who share similar passions. Whether joining a photography club, taking a cooking class, or attending a language exchange, these social interactions help expand one's social network and lead to lasting friendships.

Engaging in activities with others provides social support and reinforces a sense of community. This is particularly important today, where loneliness and social isolation are increasingly common.

2.4. Boosting Creativity and Innovation

Exploring new hobbies stimulates creativity by allowing individuals to experiment with different methods and approaches to problem-solving. Creative activities like painting, writing, or photography encourage self-expression and innovative thinking. Moreover, trying new hobbies can lead to unexpected discoveries. For example, someone who takes up digital art may find a new interest in graphic design or animation. At the same time, a person learning woodworking may develop an interest in architecture or interior design.

Creativity is essential for personal and professional development. It helps individuals think outside the box, solve problems innovatively, and express themselves authentically.

Section 3: Balancing Work, Life, and Leisure

A healthy balance between work, life, and leisure is essential for well-being. This section will explore strategies for achieving this balance and ensuring that hobbies and leisure time are not neglected.

3.1. The Importance of Time Management

Practical time management is a key component of balancing work, life, and leisure. In today's busy world, making time for hobbies and personal interests can be challenging. However, with careful planning, it is possible to prioritize personal well-being alongside work and other responsibilities.

Time management strategies such as creating schedules, setting goals, and allocating specific times for hobbies can help individuals ensure they are giving enough attention to their interests. Treating hobbies as a priority is essential, just like any other work task or responsibility. This can include setting aside certain evenings or weekends for engaging in hobbies, whether gardening, reading, or practicing a musical instrument.

3.2. Setting Boundaries and Managing Expectations

Setting boundaries is another critical aspect of balancing work, life, and leisure. In today's connected world, it is easy to constantly check emails or respond to work-related messages during personal time. Establishing boundaries around work and leisure time is crucial for ensuring that hobbies do not take a backseat.

For example, setting clear boundaries around work hours, limiting overtime, and avoiding bringing work home can create more space for personal activities. Similarly, managing family or social expectations regarding time commitments is vital to avoid burnout and resentment.

3.3. The Role of Self-Care and Leisure in Productivity

It is often said that "you can't pour from an empty cup." Taking time to engage in hobbies and relaxation is an essential form of self-care. While taking time away from work for personal leisure may seem counterintuitive, research has shown that taking breaks and engaging in relaxing activities can enhance productivity in the long run. Hobbies allow individuals to recharge mentally and emotionally, making them more focused and efficient when returning to work or responsibilities.

3.4. Integrating Hobbies into Daily Life

Incorporating hobbies into daily life is another way to ensure they remain a priority. For instance, individuals can turn their commute into a time for learning by listening to podcasts or audiobooks, or they can engage in hobbies during lunch breaks or after work. Small changes, like setting aside just 30 minutes daily for a favorite activity, can make a significant difference in maintaining a balanced lifestyle.

Conclusion

In conclusion, hobbies and personal interests are vital components of overall well-being. They provide numerous psychological, emotional, and physical benefits, from stress relief to cognitive enhancement. Exploring new interests offers opportunities for mental stimulation, creativity, and social connection while balancing work, life, and leisure, essential for maintaining a healthy lifestyle. By prioritizing hobbies and managing time effectively, individuals can create a fulfilling and balanced life that supports personal and professional growth.

Chapter 19: Creating a Personal Health Plan

Creating a personal health plan is a powerful and transformative process involving a proactive health management approach. It empowers you to prioritize your well-being, set meaningful goals, and design a pathway that enhances your physical, mental, and emotional health. Whether you're looking to improve fitness, manage stress, improve nutrition, or overcome chronic conditions, a personalized health plan allows you to take control and make deliberate, sustainable changes to your lifestyle. This chapter will delve into the key aspects of creating a personal health plan, including the steps involved in developing one, setting achievable health goals, and the importance of accountability and tracking progress.

1. **Steps to Develop a Personalized Health Plan**

Developing a personalized health plan is a structured process that requires you to reflect on your current health, set clear goals, and design a plan that aligns with your lifestyle. The steps to creating an effective health plan are:

1.1 Assessing Your Current Health Status

The first step in developing a personal health plan is to assess where you currently stand regarding your health. This involves a comprehensive review of your physical, mental, and emotional well-being. You may want to start by considering the following:

- **Physical Health**: Evaluate your fitness level, weight, body composition, and medical conditions such as hypertension, diabetes, or heart disease. Note any symptoms you may be experiencing, like fatigue, pain, or digestive issues.

- **Mental and Emotional Health**: Assess your cognitive health by assessing your mood, stress levels, anxiety, and overall mental clarity. Identify any signs of depression, burnout, or overwhelming stress. When creating a personal health plan, mental health is as important as physical health.

- **Lifestyle Factors**: Review your lifestyle habits, such as your diet, exercise routine, sleep patterns, smoking, alcohol consumption, and stress management strategies. Identify areas where improvements can be made to align your lifestyle with your health goals.

The more thorough your self-assessment is, the more precise the starting point for your personal health plan will be.

1.2 Defining Your Health Goals

Once you've assessed your current health status, the next step is to define your goals. Health goals should be specific, measurable, achievable, relevant, and time-bound (SMART). This helps ensure that your goals are clear and attainable. Goals can be divided into short-term, medium-term, and long-term categories:

- **Short-term Goals**: These are goals you can achieve in the next few weeks or months, such as reducing stress, eating more fruits and vegetables, or increasing your physical activity levels.
- **Medium-term Goals**: These goals are typically achievable within six months to a year, such as losing a specific amount of weight, improving cardiovascular health, or mastering a new workout routine.
- **Long-term Goals**: These goals require more extended time frames (over a year or more) and may involve maintaining a healthy weight, managing a chronic illness, or adopting an entirely new lifestyle.

1.3 Identifying Resources and Support

A personalized health plan doesn't have to be created in isolation. Identifying the resources and support systems that can help you achieve your health goals is essential. This might include:

- **Professional Support**: Healthcare professionals like doctors, dietitians, personal trainers, therapists, or counselors can offer valuable advice and guidance in achieving your health goals.
- **Support Systems**: Friends, family, or support groups can provide encouragement and motivation throughout your journey. Community support, such as fitness classes, online forums, or local health clubs, can also be valuable resources.
- **Tools and Resources**: Consider leveraging technology, such as fitness apps, meditation apps, or nutrition trackers, to monitor your progress. Books, podcasts, or educational courses on health topics can also be beneficial.

1.4 Creating an Action Plan

After defining your goals and identifying the resources, the next step is to create an actionable plan. Break your larger goals into smaller, manageable tasks that can be easily integrated into your daily routine. For example:

- **Daily Tasks**: These can include taking a daily walk, drinking a certain amount of water, practicing mindfulness, or tracking your food intake.

- **Weekly Tasks**: Weekly tasks might involve meal prepping, attending fitness classes, scheduling exercise sessions, or meditating for a set time.
- **Monthly Tasks**: Monthly tasks can include reviewing progress, adjusting goals if necessary, or seeking professional advice to improve.

The key is to create a realistic and sustainable plan that will gradually bring you closer to your overall health goals.

1. **Setting Achievable Health Goals**

Setting achievable health goals is crucial for long-term success. Unrealistic goals can lead to frustration and burnout, whereas setting realistic and manageable goals helps you stay motivated and makes the journey toward health improvement feel more rewarding.

2.1 Make Your Goals Specific and Clear

A vague goal like "I want to be healthier" lacks the clarity and focus needed for success. Instead, specify what "healthier" means to you. For instance, a more explicit goal might be "I want to lose 10 pounds in the next three months" or "I want to reduce my blood pressure by 10 points."

2.2 Make Your Goals Measurable

Measurable goals allow you to track your progress over time. This helps you stay motivated and shows tangible evidence of your hard work. For example, instead of setting a goal like "I want to exercise more," make it measurable by saying, "I want to exercise for 30 minutes five days a week."

2.3 Ensure Goals Are Achievable

Given your current circumstances, it's essential to set goals that are within your capabilities. While challenging yourself is crucial, setting too difficult goals can lead to failure and discouragement. For example, aiming to lose 5 pounds in a month may be realistic for some, but more than 20 pounds may be achievable quickly for most people.

2.4 Set Relevant and Meaningful Goals

Your health goals should be relevant to your needs and values. For example, if you're focused on managing a chronic condition like diabetes, your goals might center around maintaining stable blood sugar levels through diet and exercise. Setting goals that resonate with your health needs ensures you stay engaged and committed.

2.5 Establish a time frame

Setting a timeframe helps to create a sense of urgency and keeps you focused on your progress. Deadlines encourage consistency and reduce procrastination. However, these timelines must be realistic, as progress in health can often be gradual.

1. **Importance of Accountability and Tracking Progress**

Accountability and tracking progress are critical elements in achieving your health goals. They ensure that you remain motivated, make adjustments when necessary, and celebrate your successes.

3.1 The Role of Accountability in Health Plans

Accountability is about taking responsibility for your actions and progress. It provides external motivation and a sense of obligation. Here are a few ways to incorporate accountability into your health plan:

- **Accountability Partners**: Having someone to share your goals with, such as a friend, family member, or personal coach, can significantly improve your commitment. Regular check-ins with an accountability partner can help keep you on track and provide moral support during challenging times.

- **Group Challenges or Support Groups**: Participating in a fitness challenge or joining a group working toward similar health goals can foster motivation and make you feel more connected to others who understand your journey.

- **Social Media or Online Communities**: Some people find it helpful to share their progress online. Social media platforms or online health communities can provide virtual accountability; others can encourage you, share tips, or offer support.

3.2 Tracking Progress Effectively

Tracking your progress provides a clear picture of how far you've come and helps identify areas that need improvement. Regular progress checks also reinforce positive behaviors and help you stay motivated. Some practical ways to track your health progress include:

- **Daily Logs**: Keeping a journal or using a fitness app to record your activities, food intake, sleep patterns, and emotional well-being can provide valuable insights.

- **Weekly Reviews**: Take time each week to assess how well you adhere to your plan. Are you meeting your exercise and nutrition goals? Do you feel better physically and mentally?

- **Monthly Check-ins**: Set aside time at the end of each month to evaluate your overall progress. Have you made improvements in your health goals? If not, what adjustments can you make for the upcoming month?

- **Body Measurements and Health Metrics**: Regularly measuring your weight, body measurements (waist, hips, etc.), blood pressure, or blood sugar levels can give you a concrete view of your health improvements.

3.3 Adjusting Your Plan

As you track your progress, it's essential to be flexible with your health plan. If you find that certain goals are too challenging or unrealistic, you may need to adjust them. On the other hand, if you're surpassing your expectations, you may want to challenge yourself further.

Adjustments are a natural part of any health journey. Be open to changing your approach while staying focused on your overarching goals.

3.4 Celebrating Successes

Remember to celebrate the milestones and successes along the way. Whether you're losing your first 5 pounds, hitting your step goal every day for a month, or simply feeling more energized and less stressed, acknowledging these achievements boosts morale and encourages you to continue on your health journey.

Conclusion

Creating a personal health plan is an empowering way to take control of your health and well-being. You can embark on a healthier, happier life by following the steps outlined in this chapter:

- Assessing your current health
- Defining realistic and measurable goals
- Leveraging resources and support
- Ensuring accountability and progress tracking

Remember that the journey is ongoing.

Chapter 20: Inspiring Change: Real-Life Success Stories

This chapter explores the power of personal transformation through health and wellness journeys. It aims to inspire readers by showcasing the real-life stories of men who faced health challenges and transformed their lives. Through these stories, the chapter uncovers the lessons learned from these transformations, offering valuable insights, advice, and actionable encouragement to readers on the verge of embarking on their health journeys. The aim is to highlight success and foster a sense of hope and possibility for anyone willing to make a change in their life.

1. **Introduction to Personal Transformation**

Health transformations are more than just physical changes; they are deeply personal, emotional, and often life-altering experiences. This chapter opens by explaining how each individual's journey to better health is unique but united by a common thread: the decision to take control of their health. It underscores the reality that no transformation happens overnight. It takes commitment, sacrifice, and, most importantly, the belief that change is possible. The chapter introduces the importance of inspiration in the transformation process and sets the tone for the following personal stories. The intention is to make the reader feel that they can achieve meaningful change no matter their starting point.

1. **Compilation of Personal Stories from Men Who Transformed Their Health**

In this section, we explore the individual journeys of several men who have successfully improved their health. These stories come from various backgrounds and touch on mental health, weight loss, chronic illness management, fitness, nutrition, and lifestyle changes. Each story reflects the personal challenges these men faced, their turning points, and their actions to bring about change.

- **John's Weight Loss Journey**
- John, a 45-year-old corporate executive, was struggling with obesity and type 2 diabetes. He had spent years working long hours, eating unhealthy meals on the go, and neglecting his fitness. This led to a diagnosis that served as a wake-up call. His story chronicles the moment he realized that he needed to take control of his life. He began by making small changes: walking daily, tracking his food, and gradually introducing healthier meals into his routine. Through consistency and discipline, John lost 80 pounds and significantly improved his diabetes management.
- **Mark's Fight Against Heart Disease**

- Mark, 58, was diagnosed with coronary artery disease after a routine check-up. Despite a history of heart disease in his family, Mark had lived a sedentary lifestyle. His story details how he took his diagnosis seriously, changed his diet, started exercising regularly, and worked with his doctor to find the proper medications. He reversed some of the effects of his heart condition and gained a new sense of purpose by sharing his experiences with others at local health forums.
- **David's Mental Health and Fitness Journey**
- David, a 34-year-old entrepreneur, struggled with anxiety and depression, exacerbated by his demanding job. After years of battling with his mental health, David decided to try a holistic approach, combining therapy with physical activity. He found that regular exercise, especially weightlifting, significantly helped in reducing his anxiety levels and gave him more control over his emotions. His journey includes his exploration of mindfulness and nutrition and how they all intertwine to restore his sense of balance.
- **Tom's Transformation Through Plant-Based Nutrition**
- Tom, a 52-year-old teacher, had suffered from high cholesterol and frequent fatigue for years. After learning about the benefits of plant-based eating, he boldly decided to overhaul his diet completely. His story focuses on the challenges he faced in adjusting to a plant-based lifestyle, the obstacles he overcame, and how this choice helped him lose weight and feel more energetic and clear-headed.
- **Ethan's Rebuilding After Injury**
- Ethan, a 30-year-old former athlete, faced a career-ending injury that left him physically and emotionally broken. After months of physical therapy, Ethan realized that the road to recovery wasn't just about physical healing; it was about mental resilience. He embraced functional fitness and adapted his routines to rebuild his strength and regain his confidence. His story highlights the role of perseverance and the power of setting small goals that contribute to long-term progress.

1. **Lessons Learned from Their Journeys**

Each transformation story holds valuable lessons that can benefit anyone looking to make positive changes in their own lives. This section breaks down the key insights from the success stories:

- **Consistency Over Perfection**
- One common thread throughout these stories is the importance of consistency. Whether it was John losing weight, Mark managing his heart disease, or David improving his mental health, they all learned that perfection is unnecessary to make progress. Success is about showing up, day in and day out, even when motivation wanes. It's

about doing something every day, no matter how small, to move closer to your goal.

- **The Power of a Support System**
- Transformation isn't done alone. All the men in these stories emphasized the importance of a support system—be it family, friends, or a community. Support keeps you accountable, encourages you during tough times, and reminds you that you are not alone. The journey can feel overwhelming, but the right people can make all the difference.
- **Small Changes Lead to Big Results**
- Another important lesson is that small, incremental changes often lead to lasting results. In each story, the men start with minor modifications, like drinking more water, walking, or cooking a healthier meal. Over time, these small steps snowballed into larger, life-changing habits. Rather than trying to overhaul everything at once, the key takeaway is to focus on making minor adjustments that can be sustained in the long term.
- **Mindset is Everything**
- A crucial element in these transformations was the shift in mindset. The men in these stories had to change their thinking about themselves and their health. For many, it involved moving from self-doubt or complacency to empowerment and discipline. The mental and physical transformation showed that health is a holistic pursuit.
- **Personal Accountability**
- Each success story demonstrated the importance of taking responsibility for one's actions. This was especially true for men like Tom, who made a drastic diet change, and Ethan, who had to rebuild his body after an injury. The journey required them to hold themselves accountable for their choices and to take ownership of their well-being.
- **Patience and Resilience**
- Health transformation is not a quick fix; these men learned that resilience is key. There were setbacks, plateaus, and moments of doubt, but they persevered. The lesson here is that actual change takes time. Those who embraced this truth could ride out the rough patches and see lasting results in the long run.

1. **Advice for Readers: Taking Action in Their Own Lives**

The final part of this chapter encourages readers to take action in their own health journeys. Drawing inspiration from the stories and lessons shared, this section offers practical advice and strategies to help readers start on their own paths to health transformation.

- **Start Small, But Start Now**

- Don't wait for the "perfect" moment to begin your transformation. Start with something manageable, whether walking for 10 minutes daily or cutting out one unhealthy food item from your diet. The key is to start today, not tomorrow.
- **Set Realistic Goals**
- Define what success looks like for you, but make sure your goals are achievable. Set both short-term and long-term goals, and celebrate each small victory along the way. Remember, it's about progress, not perfection.
- **Seek Help When Needed**
- Feel free to ask for help. The right guidance can make a world of difference in your journey, whether you hire a personal trainer, join a support group, or consult with a healthcare professional.
- **Focus on the Why**
- Understand your reasons for wanting to make a change. Whether improving your health, gaining energy, or simply feeling better in your skin, knowing your "why" will keep you motivated when challenges arise.
- **Build a Routine**
- Consistency is key. Build a routine incorporating the habits that will help you succeed, and stick to it as much as possible. The more it becomes part of your daily life, the less you'll need to rely on willpower to stay on track.
- **Celebrate Your Wins**
- Take time to acknowledge your progress, no matter how small it may seem. Celebrating your victories, whether losing a few pounds, improving your stamina, or feeling mentally clearer, reinforces positive behavior and motivates you to continue.

1. **Conclusion: The Power of Change**

The chapter concludes by reinforcing the power of transformation. Each man's story highlights the idea that change is not just possible; it's achievable. By starting small, building momentum, and staying consistent, anyone can overcome the obstacles that prevent them from living their healthiest life. The stories in this chapter are meant to be a source of motivation and a reminder that with effort and perseverance, success is within reach. Readers are encouraged to reflect on their own health and wellness goals, armed with inspiration from those who have walked the path before them. The journey to better health is not just about the destination. It's about who you become along the way.

Conclusion

Congratulations! By reading Men's Health Unlocked: A Guide to Living Well, you've taken an essential first step toward prioritizing your health and well-being. This journey is not about quick fixes or one-size-fits-all solutions; it's about creating a sustainable, lifelong commitment to becoming the best version of yourself physically and mentally.

As you've learned throughout this book, achieving optimal health involves a balanced approach that includes:

- **Regular physical activity** that challenges your body and enhances your fitness.
- **Proper nutrition** fuels you with the energy and nutrients needed for everyday success.
- **Mental well-being practices** that help you manage stress and cultivate emotional resilience.
- **Healthy lifestyle choices** that focus on rest, relationships, and self-care for long-term health.

Your Health is a Lifelong Journey

Health is not a destination. It's an ongoing journey. The small, consistent steps you take daily compound to create significant, lasting change. Whether you've already started implementing some of the strategies in this book or are just beginning, remember that progress is made through persistence, not perfection. Setbacks are natural and part of the process, so don't let them discourage you. Instead, see them as opportunities to learn, grow, and adjust. Every step you take, no matter how small, moves you closer to a healthier, more fulfilling life.

Keep Moving Forward

Please take what you've learned here and put it into practice. Whether it's adjusting your diet, committing to regular exercise, or setting aside time for mental relaxation, the key is consistency. Celebrate your wins, big or small, and be bold and revisit the strategies in this book whenever you need a boost. You have the power to shape your health and your future. Make that choice today, and continue unlocking your best self. Here's to a future of strength, vitality, and well-being.

Thank you for reading, and best of luck on your journey to better health!

Thank You

www.ingramcontent.com/pod-product-compliance
Lightning Source LLC
Chambersburg PA
CBHW051829250726

48659CB00005B/1745